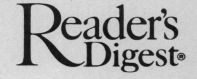

FAMILY SAFETY
& FIRST AID

THE EDITORS OF *READER'S DIGEST*

A BERKLEY/READER'S DIGEST BOOK
published by
BERKLEY BOOKS, NEW YORK

READER'S DIGEST FAMILY SAFETY & FIRST AID

A Berkley/Reader's Digest Book / published by arrangement with
Reader's Digest Press

PRINTING HISTORY
Berkley/Reader's Digest trade paperback edition / June 1984
Second printing / January 1985

ISBN: 0-425-06817-X

Reader's Digest Paperbacks

Informative . . . . . Entertaining . . . . . Essential . . . . .

Berkley, one of America's leading paperback publishers, is proud to present this special series of the best-loved articles, stories and features from America's most trusted magazine. Each is a one-volume library on a popular and important subject. And each is selected, edited and endorsed by the Editors of Reader's Digest themselves!

READER'S DIGEST FAMILY SAFETY & FIRST AID is not designed to eliminate the need for a physician when complex problems arise, but to help you understand your situation should you have to consult a doctor. Throughout, the book emphasizes the truth of the saying that what you don't know about safety and first aid *can* hurt you.

Why you need medical or safety advice. FAMILY SAFETY & FIRST AID is not a substitute for a professional opinion. No single book dealing with the number of topics discussed in FAMILY SAFETY & FIRST AID could state the individual applications of safety and first aid principles. What FAMILY SAFETY & FIRST AID does tell you is the basics of safety and first aid. This book is not intended as a substitute for a doctor, however, nor as a do-it-yourself first aid kit. It does suggest when you may or may not require a physician's services. But in any serious situation, or when you are in doubt, there is no substitute for competent professional advice. Trying to act as your own doctor or safety expert can be costly and—in some instances—dangerous.

Contents

PART ONE: SAFETY BEGINS AT HOME

Chapter One—Is Your House a Death Trap?

The Most Dangerous Place in the World—Your House   3
Help For House Hazards   7
Death in the Kitchen   11
A Little Box That Stops Electric Shock   14
Beware Those Holiday Accidents   18
Cut the Grass—Not Yourself!   22

Chapter Two—Protect Your Children

Can't We Stop These Tragic Injuries to Children?   27
When Children Are in the Car   32

Chapter Three—Poison: Handle With Care

Home Canning: The Safe Way   39
Food Poisoning—And How to Avoid It   45
"Help! My Child Has Taken Poison!"   49
Postscript: Home Treatment For Poisoning   54

Chapter Four—House Fire!

Is Your Home a Family Firetrap?   **57**
ESDs—Those Astonishing Little Fire Alarms   **63**

PART TWO: SAFETY OUTSIDE THE HOME

Chapter Five—How to Stay Safe Outdoors

What To Do When Lightning Strikes   **71**
Danger! Stinging Insects   **75**
Sunbathing—In a New Light   **77**

Chapter Six—Safety in the Water

Secrets To Not Drowning in the Sea   **85**
"Rescue Breathing"—The Way to Save Lives   **90**
Cold Can Do You In   **93**
Boating Safety Is No Accident   **97**
Your Spare Tire Can Prevent a Drowning   **103**

Chapter Seven—Safety Away From Home

Traveling in Good Health   **109**
Hitchhiking—Too Often the Last Ride   **113**
Is Your Child's School Safe From Fire?   **118**

Chapter Eight—Some Environmental Hazards

Watch Out For Electric Smog   **125**
Warning: X Rays May Be Dangerous to Your Health   **130**

PART THREE: STAYING ALIVE ON THE ROAD

Chapter Nine—Principles of Safe Driving

How to Stay Alive on the Highways   **137**
Tailgating—Invitation to Tragedy   **141**
How to Fight Highway Hypnosis   **145**
Marijuana and Driving: The Sobering Truth   **149**

Can You "Talk" to Other Drivers?   **155**
Twelve Suggestions for Safer Driving   **159**

Chapter Ten–Driving In Hazardous Conditions

Ten Tips For Winter Driving   **163**
How to Drive in Fog   **166**
Pills Drivers Shouldn't Take   **168**
How to Drive Out of Trouble   **172**

Chapter Eleven–Danger On Two Wheels

Safety-First For Cyclists   **179**
Moped Madness   **183**

PART FOUR: FIRST AID

Chapter Twelve–Be Prepared

The Tag That Can Save Your Life   **189**
Are You Accident-Prone?   **193**
How Quick-Witted Are You?   **198**

Chapter Thirteen–An Ounce of Prevention

Heed Your Body's Warning Signals   **203**
Six Ways to Reduce Your Cancer Risk   **208**
What You Should Know About Eye Care   **209**
Danger, Danger, Everywhere   **215**
A Do-It-Yourself Health Check-Up   **220**

Chapter Fourteen–How to Cope With an Emergency

How to Recognize—and Survive—a Heart Attack   **229**
CPR—The Lifesaving Technique Everyone Should Know   **236**
Snakebite: The Forgotten Menace   **240**
The Heimlich Maneuver: Help the Choking Victim   **245**

READER'S DIGEST HANDBOOK OF FIRST AID   **247**

PART ONE
SAFETY BEGINS AT HOME

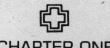

CHAPTER ONE

IS YOUR HOUSE A DEATH TRAP?

The Most Dangerous Place In the World— Your House

by Albert Q. Maisel

IN THE TIME it will take you to read this article, 435 of your fellow Americans will suffer injuries in their own homes. By this time tomorrow 63,000 of us will have cut, bruised, scalded, burned or poisoned ourselves—at home. In the next year about nine million of us will have had to call a doctor to tend our home injuries, and 3.4 million of us will have been disabled—laid up at least a day. Twenty-three thousand of us will have died from falls, burns, poisons, suffocation, or as a result of other accidents suffered while "safe" at home.

And the figures are mounting. To the booby traps that have always existed in our homes—the torn carpet, the dark staircase, the toys left scattered on the floor—mechanization has added whole new categories of accident-inviting hazards.

As we install more and more appliances, overloaded wiring systems touch off increasing thousands of fires.

Do-it-yourselfism, insurance men report, results in 600,000 injuries a year. We fall from roofs and ladders, mash and lacerate ourselves with power tools. In one recent year, hospital emergency rooms had to treat more than 70,000 persons injured by their power mowers.

Behind these figures stand two arresting facts.

• Most of our 23 million annual home accidents need never happen at all. They are the result either of plain carelessness or of failure to eliminate hazards that could easily have been foreseen.

• Millions of the victims of these accidents suffer needless pain and disability—and some, in fact, die—because no one on the scene knows what kind of first aid to give once they are hurt.

But *your* house, you think, is a pretty safe place. I thought mine was, too—until my wife challenged me to join her in a thorough check. We ended our tour chastened. Everywhere we found hazards that should have been corrected long ago: 20 in the house alone and nearly a dozen others in the garage and on the grounds.

Check your own house—and habits—against the following safety list:

Is your TV set or hi-fi properly ventilated? Manufacturers provide adequate ventilation in their cabinets, but the heat of tubes in sets that have been re-enclosed in built-in units accounts for scores of home fires.

Are there enough ashtrays—big enough ones—the kind that won't let a forgotten cigarette fall out onto upholstery or rugs?

Is your fireplace screen stable? Do you always close the screen before leaving the house or retiring?

Are firearms kept in locked cabinets?

Are lamp cords free of frayed spots? Are they short enough not to become tangled and trip people?

Do you make it a rule never to smoke in bed? Approximately 500 Americans cremate themselves that way every year.

Are perfumes, cosmetics, needles, pins, scissors, spare buttons kept out of your children's reach?

Can everyone—children and old people especially—reach a light switch *before* getting out of bed?

Do youngsters put toys away before going to bed so that their bedroom floors are left uncluttered?

Are knives and other sharp implements stored separately out of children's reach?

Are detergents, polishes, bleaches, drain solvents, spot removers and other toxic chemicals stored in high cabinets or locked compartments? Over 12 percent of all accidental poisonings are caused by cleaning and sanitizing compounds.

Do you always keep pot handles turned away from the stove edge so that pots cannot be accidentally overturned? Is your water-heater thermostat set too high? Kitchen burns and scalds kill many persons every year, inflict pain and permanent scars on thousands of others.

Do you have an *adequate* first-aid kit? We found the antiseptic in ours evaporated, the bandages in a tangle and the scissors rusted shut.

Do you keep dangerous drugs in a cabinet children can't open? (All drugs should be considered dangerous if youngsters can get at them. Aspirin, for instance, is responsible for one accidental poisoning in every 40 among children under five.)

Is there a grab bar above your tub and in the shower stall? And a rubber mat at the bottom of each? Are light switches far enough away so that they cannot be operated by anyone standing in tub or shower?

Are you using 20- or 25-ampere fuses in circuits that are wired for 15 amperes?

Are the cellar stairs well lighted, with a switch *outside* the entrance door? Do they have secure handrails?

Are your tools locked away or out of reach? Are power tools always disconnected when not in use? Have you disposed of oil-soaked rags, piles of old clothes, newspapers and other refuse that might start or feed a fire?

Have your furnace, chimney and flues been cleaned within the last year?

Do you store insecticides, rodent poisons, weed killers, etc., in a locked cabinet in the garage or tool shed?

Are clotheslines strung high enough so that no one can run into them?

Is your garage free of old paint cans, rusting tools, bottles, nails, garden stakes?

Do you insist that others leave the lawn when you operate your rotary power mower?

Have you equipped your garage (and kitchen) with fire extinguishers labeled by the Underwriters or Factory Mutual Laboratories?

MILLIONS of us couldn't honestly claim even a near-passing grade on this home-safety test. And along with our failure to observe the simplest precautions goes an equally astonishing lack of basic common sense in our handling of injuries.

Tourniquets, for example, should be used only in an extreme emergency, when all other methods to control bleeding have failed, and only by those with special training. Instead, they are sometimes applied by frightened first-aiders and then left tight until the limb turns blue from lack of circulating blood. So frequent is this error that many hospitals instruct their ambulance and emergency-room attendants to loosen the tourniquet as soon as they have applied pressure to the wound.

Another common error that aggravates injuries is the smearing of burns with greasy ointments or even with butter or lard. Then, when a physician is called, he has to deal not only with a burn but possibly with infection as well.

Delays in seeking professional treatment are widespread. Doctors often have to treat day-old ankle fractures complicated by excessive swelling, because both the injured and those who aided them assumed that they were dealing with nothing worse than a sprain.

The opposite mistake, moving a person with a broken neck or back, is equally common. The result? Almost always a delayed recovery and sometimes a totally unnecessary death.

How can you best protect yourself and your family against such disasters?

Your first step, obviously, is to eliminate every physical hazard you can recognize in and around your home and to keep checking for new hazards every month or so.

Next, train and drill every member of your household to avoid the unsafe acts that combine with unsafe conditions to produce accidents. Repeat the drill periodically, the way a school repeats its fire drills, until safe conduct becomes second nature.

Finally, since *all* accidents cannot possibly be foreseen and prevented, bone up on first aid and insist that the other members of your family do, too.

A time-consuming program? Yes. It may mean spending five or even ten hours a year. But is that too big a price to pay to ward off months of pain, crippling—and, maybe, needless death?

Help For House Hazards

by Goody L. Solomon

EACH YEAR, American homes are the scene of about 3.4 *million* reported disabling injuries from accidents, resulting in $8.9 billion in lost work time, medical bills, insurance administrative costs and fire loss. Many injuries that require emergency room treatment involve structural components of houses: glass doors and windows inflict about 200,000 injuries; tubs and showers, 77,000; stairs, 750,000.

Most home accidents result from a mix of human error and hazardous surroundings. While humans will always make mistakes, there *are* things you can do to make key areas in your home safer. For example:

Plumbing and fixtures

Water heated to 115° can injure human skin; yet most water heaters are set at 140° to 160°. Lowering the heater thermostat to 115° reduces the hazard, but it also produces water insufficiently hot for some dishwashers and washing machines. The remedy is a thermostatic valve or blender, which may cost $100 or more and can be fitted onto the water heater, for a plumber's fee of $40 to $50 more. As hot water leaves the heater, the valve mixes cold water into it so it won't scald. Lines bypassing the valve supply appliances that need really hot water.

Even a slippery bathtub can be rendered safer. Paste no-skid stickers on the bottom—a set of ten costs only $3.20—or use a $3.50 rubber

7

mat. When buying a new tub, consider one made of fiberglass. Its resilience provides more secure footing and softens a fall. Tubs with embossed bottoms have come on the market as a safety innovation; but, according to some safety specialists, soap scum may accumulate in the indentations. Therefore these, as well as tub stickers, should be kept clean of soap scum.

Other tips for safer bathrooms:

• Install grab bars within the confines of tubs and showers.

• Cover glazed-tile floors, preferably with wall-to-wall carpeting.

Stairs

Going up or down steps is one of the most dangerous things a person does in a house. The most effective countermeasure: install handrails. Almost anybody can make one—it takes $3 worth of brackets and a length of railing, which costs about $3.50 a foot.

Some stairways are risky because their treads are narrow, their risers steep. Either condition calls for a new staircase. A straight pine staircase one story high may cost between $400 and $600 (installed).

Basement stairs often combine two dangers: no landing platform at the top, and a door that opens out over the stairway. The climber must step down backward to open it, and a person coming the other way may not be prepared for the sudden change in floor level. The stairs ought to be rebuilt to provide a landing wide enough to accommodate the full swing of the door. At a minimum, the door should be rehung to open away from the climber, or to fold or slide. An accordion-type door may cost $75 if it's plastic, $170 or more if it's wood.

Other precautions for stairs:

• Some basement stairways have handrails with a single center support pole midway down the open side; anyone can fall through to the hard floor below. The stairs can be enclosed with decorative wrought iron, additional wood supports, peg board or paneling.

• Poor lighting and shadows contribute to many accidents on stairs. Install switches at both top and bottom, and reduce the glare by using frosted bulbs.

• Slippery wooden treads are another cause of stairway accidents. They should be covered. Carpeting for the average stairway will run

$210 to $250 installed; a runner allows some wood to show and costs about $120. For basement or attic stairs, consider a coat of paint or varnish to add friction.

The electrical system

One household risk may be aluminum wiring. Generally between 1965 and 1973, electricians put aluminum wire (cheaper than the more traditional copper) into an estimated two million houses and into many repair jobs. According to the U.S. Consumer Product Safety Commission, aluminum can work loose from connections, generating heat as current is forced through the resultant poor connection, and when this happens, fire is a possibility.

If *your* wiring is aluminum—or if you think it may be but aren't sure—you should:

• Write or call the U.S. Consumer Product Safety Commission, Washington, D.C. 20207.

• Call an electrician if you find a switch or receptacle that feels warm, if you smell hot or burning plastic near an outlet or switch, or if lights flicker inexplicably.

Doors and windows

A visitor knocks on a door pane and his hand goes through the glass; a youngster rides his tricycle through the storm door; a woman runs to answer the telephone and crashes through the patio door; a bather slips in the tub and crashes against the glass enclosure.

Such accidents aren't rare; in fact, the federal government now requires safety glazing for new and replacement panes in entrance and exit doors, in storm doors and bath enclosures. Rigid plastic, tempered glass, and laminated glass are considered safe. Tempered glass has five times the strength of ordinary glass. When it breaks, it disintegrates into small pieces resembling rock salt instead of long razor-sharp shards. Laminated glass, used in car windshields, is a sandwich of glass with a filler of tough vinyl. Laminated glass breaks more easily than tempered glass, but it won't shatter. Rigid plastic is hardest to break, but it gets scratched, and some cleaning compounds may turn it yellow or make it hazy.

A full-length patio-door pane may cost about $130 in tempered glass, $160 in plastic, and $35 in laminated glass, not including installation. (A less-expensive safety scheme is the application of decorative decals to call attention to the glass.)

Another way to avoid injury is to put stops on swinging doors, so that they can swing in only one direction.

Death
in the Kitchen

by Louis I. Dublin, Ph.D. with Molly Castle

IN THE kitchen, moving about from counter to stove to sink, the housewife goes her perilous way quite unaware of the dangers that constantly beset her. The kitchen is the most lethal room in your house. Thousands of persons die each year from injuries sustained in the kitchen; hundreds more die as the result of gas, fire and other hazards which have their origin there; and many times that number suffer serious injuries.

Kitchen burns and scalds prove fatal for many persons every year, and for each one killed a hundred others are permanently or temporarily disabled. But there are also those who are poisoned, electrocuted or gassed. People fall or slip, get mangled or cut, or blow themselves up.

One of the most obvious, yet frequently neglected, precautions is to keep pan handles from jutting out over the edge of the stove. These can be caught in the clothing and pulled off, or a toddler may grasp at a handle above his head and tip over himself a pan of boiling water or hot grease.

Each year hundreds lose their lives or are seriously burned while cleaning with flammable fluids. Cleaning fluid evaporates, and the fumes of flammable ones are readily ignited by the pilot light of a gas stove, or by a cigarette or a distant flame.

Falls in the home, many of which occur in the kitchen, are responsible for about 6500 kitchen deaths a year. Spilled grease or soapy water can make a kitchen floor as slippery as a ski slide. Many a fracture is the result of wet or improperly waxed floors, or worn floor covering. Otherwise sane people often will try to reach top shelves by way of precarious devices—and suffer bad falls.

Cuts from kitchen knives, broken glass and china, sharp cans or peeling tools are probably the most frequent kitchen accidents. Usually they are not fatal.

Death comes a good deal sooner than it need to those who overlook the mechanics of the gas range or the principles of electricity. The ordinary household current can kill. The danger is multiplied when wet hands turn a switch or pull out wall plugs. Young children have died from putting extension cords in their mouths.

Here are some kitchen cautions for your protection:

For home dry cleaning, use a nonflammable cleaning fluid, and use it outdoors or with the windows open to prevent poisoning by toxic fumes.

Keep nonedible substances (paint, cleaners, bleaches, pest poisons) out of children's reach, and in a place where they will not be mistaken for food by a hurried cook.

Keep knives in a rack from which you can take them by the handle, rather than in a drawer where you must fumble among the blades.

Never touch interior parts of electric sockets. Avoid touching any metal part of a lamp or other electrical device in such damp locations as kitchens, bathrooms, or laundries. It might be live.

Handle appliance cords carefully, and have them replaced at once when you notice a break in the insulation.

In buying any electrical or gas appliance, insist on a model that has been inspected and listed by a recognized testing laboratory. Ask for instructions on its safe use, and follow them.

Don't work near a stove while wearing loose clothes which may catch fire.

Many a fire is started by a stove left on when the phone or doorbell rings. Pressure cookers and food processors, while excellent for saving time, have to be used properly if they are not to explode or cause steam burns or cuts by being carelessly opened.

Kitchens should be planned so that they are safe in the first place; unsafe conditions must be corrected. A kitchen—especially a modern efficient one—can be fun. A funeral never is.

A Little Box
That Stops
Electric Shock

by Edward Fales, Jr.

RAIN flooded the streets of Cherry Hill, N.J., one day in August. By 5 p.m. Norman E. Toothman was worrying about his neighbors' basement. They were away, and he had promised to keep an eye on the place. He crossed the street to check.

An hour later, when he had failed to come home, his wife went to the neighbors' looking for him. She found an extension cord plugged into a kitchen outlet and leading down the basement stairs. There, lying in an inch of water on the floor beside a sump pump, was her husband, dead—electrocuted, the coroner later said, when with wet hands he plugged the cord into the pump. Current shot through him to the wet floor and into the ground.

Electric shock kills about 1000 Americans each year, nearly 300 of them in or around their homes. Thousands more will be injured, with burns or broken bones.

In Taylorsville, N.C., the Rev. Wayne Hendren was electrocuted while using a drill to repair his boat; he was sitting on an inner tube in the water. In New Hampshire, a woman died when she climbed out of her backyard pool to connect the electric water filter to an extension cord, which ran from her house. In Pierce, Neb., 15-month-old Maureen Uecker died when her tiny fingers touched the prongs of a loosely inserted light plug as she crawled across a metal furnace register. The current ran through her via the furnace to the ground. Thousands of people are injured each year by mishaps with wall sockets and extension cords alone.

Responding to an obvious need, several companies have manufactured an ingenious little box that can go a long way toward ending electric shock around the house, and even outdoors. It's called a ground fault circuit interrupter, or GFI. Suppose that you touch a faulty appliance and electricity starts to flow through your body to the ground: the little box senses the flow instantly and switches off the current. You may feel a slight shock, but it's not enough to hurt a healthy person.

How do the GFIs work? When you plug an appliance in and turn it on, the current flows in and out of the appliance over two wires, one "hot," the other "grounded" or neutral. If you touch the hot wire, or if it is in contact with the metal frame of the appliance, electricity will try to leak off through you to the ground. The amount that goes through you depends on how good a contact you make. It may be only a slight shock if you're dry-handed or standing on a dry rug, for dry skin has high electrical resistance. But if your skin is wet, or if you're standing on a damp floor or touching a gas pipe or something in contact with the ground, the current will flash through your body and into the ground— and you may be electrocuted.

It takes very little current to hurt you. For example: a flow of more than 15 amperes is necessary to blow the average household fuse; but it may take only .01 ampere to .03 to produce muscular contractions so violent that an adult cannot let go of the power source. Such shock, if long continued, can lead to asphyxiation, heart fatigue and, ultimately, death. It may take only .05 to .15 ampere to produce ventricular fibrillation, and a relatively small amount can also paralyze respiration. Larger amperages flowing through the body can produce fatal burns in internal organs.

Fuses and circuit breakers can never detect such small runaway currents. A properly built GFI can. It constantly monitors the amount of current flowing in a circuit. If there is a leakage—even a few thousandths of an ampere—the GFI's complicated electronic circuitry senses the difference and switches the electricity off. It acts within a few thousandths of a second, less than a single heartbeat, before any damage can be done.

Thus, once inserted into a circuit, a GFI can hover like a guardian angel over small children who poke forks into toasters and wives who wear an electric hair drier while washing dishes. A GFI could have saved 14-year-old Dean Holder of Costa Mesa, Calif., who was electrocuted as he sat in a metal chair in his backyard playing his electric guitar. And Mrs. Jennie Rhinehart of Ord, Neb., who touched the inside of the light socket in her refrigerator while cleaning the box. And Mrs. Harold Johnson of Haven, Kan., who stepped on a furnace grating while using a vacuum cleaner.

GFIs don't protect against the simple "line to line" short circuit— as in a frayed iron cord that sizzles and "shorts out." But in these cases, current is flowing from one wire to another in such volume that the standard household fuse or circuit breaker should blow, preventing further damage. And GFIs aren't ordinarily needed if electrical tools and appliances are properly grounded in some other way—if their cords have three-pronged plugs (the third prong being a ground connection) and these are inserted in grounded three-prong receptacles. Even here, however, a GFI can give backup protection.

The search for a GFI that would be effective for American conditions started two decades ago, when people began to build home swimming pools with underwater lights, electric pumps and filters, and poolside barbecues. Soon many swimmers were getting shocks, and the National Electric Code Committee, which sets the guidelines for municipal safety standards, began getting casualty reports.

Several makes of GFI were developed at almost the same time, all born of near-tragedy. On a vacation trip, manufacturer-inventor A. Lee Moore of South Bend, Ind., hooked his auto trailer to the electric system in a trailer park. Some insulation had rubbed off a wire inside, exposing it to the metal trailer, and when Moore's eight-year-old granddaughter touched the door, she was knocked unconscious for two hours. Moore resolved to invent a device that would prevent shock.

In Lincoln, R.I., a young engineer, J. P. Marino, was hurled across his basement while using an electric drill. He lived, but was astounded at the violence of electric shock. "It was like being run over by a truck," he says. He, too, began developing a shock-preventing device.

Meanwhile, at the University of California, Prof. Charles F. Dalziel was also working on a GFI. His interest dated back to 1920. As a Boy Scout he had built a two-mile, five-party telephone line. Somehow 120-volt electricity got into the system. It gave Dalziel a shock. And when he attempted to cut the wire, he found himself frozen to it. He tore free, but never forgot the terrible experience.

Dalziel's GFI was the first to hit the market, in 1965, mainly for use at swimming pools. A number of companies began marketing some sort of GFI in 1968, ranging from large industrial units down to shoebox-size portables that can be carried anywhere you want protection—say outdoors with electric barbecues, hedgetrimmers or Christmas lights. Now there are receptacles with GFIs built in.

Today, GFIs are required in most localities as interrupters around swimming pools and in bathrooms and garages. And prices have come down.

Beware
Those Holiday Accidents

by James H. Winchester

CHRISTMAS, which should be the most joyous of seasons, is actually the most dangerous time of the year. More home accidents occur in the United States in December than in any other month: one fatality every 19 minutes; a disabling mishap every eight seconds. The holidays are, therefore, a good time to be especially wary.

In 1969, on Christmas Day, in Saginaw, Mich., seven-year-old Dick could hardly wait to test his new dart set. With Peter, his four-year-old brother, he raced to the family garage, tacked up the small bull's-eye target, and began throwing. Suddenly he shouted, "Look out!" but it was too late. Peter, all excited, was already in the path of the six-inch-long dart with its steel needle point. The sight in his left eye is lost for life.

One of the gifts showered on 13-month-old Eugene was a musical toy. His father suspended it from two strong strings, stretched from either side of the crib, so Gene could grab it for play. But, left alone while the family ate, the active child somehow tangled the cords around his neck. Later, his mother's screams shattered the home's holiday happiness. The medical examiner's report: "Accidental hanging."

Alice, like all little girls, loves to play house, and one of Santa's gifts was a miniature electric stove. Her mother helped her prepare a cake batter, watched as Alice plugged in the connection, then left her alone in the kitchen. Looking to see how her cake was doing, Alice accidentally touched the inside of the oven—where the temperature reached 660 degrees F. Her hand received such a serious third-degree burn that she was unable to use it for weeks.

Over 3.5 billion dollars' worth of toys are sold in the United States each Christmas. Most accidents involving toys occur not because of faulty manufacture but because playthings are not appropriate to the age, interest, training, or physical capabilities of those using them. Be sure a child is old enough for the gift he gets—and remember that games like darts, suitable for older children, become real risks when smaller youngsters join the play.

Any plaything that can be broken apart is a threat to an infant or small child. Tiny pieces, such as wheels, bells, or glass and plastic eyes, can sometimes be torn off toys and swallowed. The wires and pins with which some parts are loosely attached become deadly daggers in infant hands. The wheels of wooden toys should be attached with screws, not nails.

If you must choose an electrical item, select only those which have the UL (Underwriters Laboratories) seal. (Alice's miniature stove didn't.)

Look for good construction. Arnold B. Elkind, who was chairman of the two-year President's National Commission on Product Safety, warned: "The shoddy, inexpensive toy you buy may be the most expensive gift you will ever give."

In 1969, when John, a 42-year-old father of three, began putting up his outdoor Christmas lights, he perched on a long ladder placed against the house. Suddenly the ladder slipped on the frozen ground, and he tumbled. He was laid up for weeks with a broken leg.

If there's climbing or reaching to be done, do *not* stand on a chair, table or overturned bucket. Use a sturdy ladder in good repair. John's disaster could have been averted if his ladder had had spiked feet that could be anchored firmly. Also, the foot of the ladder should be set away from the wall one fourth the distance to the upper point of support. If that is 16 feet high, set the ladder's base four feet from the wall.

Tripping or slipping sends more people to the hospital than any other home accident. Never place decorations, on the lawn or in the house, where they can trip you. Keep extension cords out of the way, presents and wrappings off the floor. Give the children a box for their toys. Follow this 3-Cs motto of the Council on Family Health: "Keep Christmas Clutter Clear."

In the middle of the night just before Christmas, while the family was in bed, sparks from a short circuit in a string of colored lights set fire to a tree in a Los Angeles home. Paper-wrapped gifts piled under the tree fed the blaze. Flames and smoke spread quickly. By the time firemen arrived, eight people were dead.

In a Cincinnati, Ohio, home, three long extension cords snaked out of a multiple-plug socket in a wall. One was connected to the Christmas-tree lights, another to a large imitation candle on the mantel, the third to a lighted Yule wreath in a front window. Together, they demanded more electricity than the normal house wiring provided.

When the fuse, in its cellar box, kept burning out—warning of a dangerous overload—the homeowner foolishly replaced it with a copper penny. This let excessive amounts of electricity go directly into the line upstairs. Not designed for the load, the wire became overheated all along its length through the walls. Result: a costly fire.

Using proper circuits and heavy-enough extension cords is a vital step toward electrical responsibility. The higher the amperage needed and the longer the cord, the larger the wire in the extension must be. (The average small string of lights handles about 1½ amperes, but people often connect several strings to one cord.)

If extensive holiday lighting is planned, call in a competent electrician to make sure that the house circuits can handle the load. Christmas lights and extension cords should be carefully inspected for loose sockets and plugs, broken wires, or insulation. (Those stored in a hot attic between Christmases may be brittle and cracked.) Never drape metallic tinsel near an electric socket. It can cause a short circuit if the two come in contact. Trains and other electrical toys which might give off a spark should be kept away from the tree. Unplug all decorative lights when they are unattended.

Advises the National Safety Council: "Hang outdoor lights with the sockets turned down, so that water won't accumulate in them and cause shorts. Make sure the UL tag is on all strings of lights themselves, not just on the box in which they're sold."

Electric lights should never be placed on metallic-foil Christmas trees. If electricity should seep from a defective cord or plug, the entire setup could become a deadly booby-trap for anyone who touched it. Off-the-tree spotlights or floodlights are recommended.

Firs, cedars and pines dry out quickly after being cut. The smallest spark or overheating can set them ablaze, and they are explosively fast burners. For this reason, many cities now restrict the use of real Christmas trees in schools, hospitals, churches and other public places. Synthetic trees made of plastic-like material burn almost as fast, unless they are flame-retardant. Artificial trees, made of aluminum or other metallic foil, are fire-resistant and safe if you avoid electrical trimmings. For those who still prefer a natural tree, buy a fresh one with springy branches and green, tight needles. Pick the tree up by the trunk and gently bump it against the ground. If many needles fall, it is too dry.

Leave your tree outside your home or in a cold place, standing in a pail of water until time to set it up. Inside, use a water stand for the tree, and keep it filled. Make sure the tree is not located near a fireplace, radiator, stove, television set or any other source of heat.

Don't leave the tree up too long. The best advice: Put it up two days before Christmas and take it down on New Year's Day. If the needles begin to drop early, get rid of it. Never burn it in the fireplace.

Christmas is a season when children, filled with excitement and intent on fun, career into sharp-edged furniture or plunge head-on into glass doors. Wanting to show off new gifts to friends, they dash across streets without looking. They can't wait to try out new toys, such as skates or bicycles, without taking the time to learn how to use them safely.

For adults, there is more than the usual amount of partying. If you are drinking, take a taxi or get someone who hasn't been drinking to drive you. If you must drive, limit yourself to about one drink per hour. If you are giving the party, casually close the bar an hour before you expect your guests to leave. Offer coffee or soft drinks for that final "one for the road."

The National Safety Council gives this summary warning: "Slow down at Christmas. Avoid doing too many things at once. Try to keep the kids from getting *too* excited. A safe Christmas starts with you."

Cut the Grass— Not Yourself!

by Paul W. Kearney

IN KANSAS City, Mo., a man lost the two middle fingers of one hand when he tried to pull some matted grass from the whirling blades of his power mower.

In Corpus Christi, Texas, a 13-year-old girl kicked at a power mower which her cousin playfully pushed toward her—and lost all the toes on her left foot.

In Collegeville, Pa., a woman was struck in the throat by the flying blade from a rotary machine which had hit an obstruction. She died before help could be obtained.

Culled from hundreds of similar mowing accidents reported in a two-week period, these casualties show why power mowers should be treated with far more wary respect than they have been so far. A study in the 1950s by the American Mutual Liability Insurance Co. disclosed that power mowers were involved in 35,000 accidents a year. When the company repeated the study some years later it was found that the casualty toll had doubled. Lost in the carnage were 50,000 toes and 18,000 fingers. Nearly a third of the victims were innocent bystanders. Yet the study clearly indicated that only some nine percent of the mishaps could be charged to true mechanical failure.

Although the power-driven reel mower was involved in part of the trouble, the less expensive and more popular rotary type was the chief offender. The rotary blade, whirling up to 200 miles per hour, is as potentially lethal as a power saw, and should be handled accordingly. Yet we do some pretty outlandish things with our rotary mowers.

Housewives often trundle rotary mowers in flimsy, open-toed sandals, when a millworker's steel-toed safety shoes and a catcher's shin guards would be more appropriate. Spiked or cleated golf shoes could well be used for grass cutting. Many accidents occur when leather soles become slippery from the grass, especially on slopes or in damp weather.

Pulling a power mower backward is dangerous because it can so easily roll over the foot. And starting a self-propelled machine while it is in gear has caused no end of misery. Even when it is out of gear, one should secure a solid, well-balanced footing, keeping the feet safely away from the undercarriage.

It must be absent-mindedness that allows mature men to pull grass out of the machine or to try to refuel or oil it while the engine is running. Quite as dangerous is refueling while the engine is still hot; a red-hot exhaust pipe can cause an explosion. Before attempting any such job, shut off the engine and wait for it to cool. Always disconnect the spark-plug wire before cleaning or making any adjustments.

Beginners make the mistake of not familiarizing themselves with the controls before using the mower. When the machine strays off course toward the flower bed, the neophyte instinctively tries to hold it back instead of instantly throwing out the clutch. When a 2½-h.p. engine has the bit in its teeth, somebody is likely to get hurt.

A major source of grief is our proclivity for taking a power mower over the lawn or into jungles of grass and weeds without first "casing" the area. A Massachusetts woman suffered cruelly lacerated legs when her rotary picked up a short length of rusty barbed wire and whipped it around her shins. An Indiana man ran over a croquet wicket, cutting it in half. One piece drilled into his leg like an arrow.

To forestall similar accidents, walk the ground before starting work—*each time you mow.* In tall weeds and "rough," drag a rake behind you as an improvised "mine detector."

Maneuvering a heavy mower on a bank or terrace is the riskiest aspect of lawn care, definitely not recommended for apprentices or for people who are not strong. Two persons can do it better than one. Enlist a helper to walk along the top of the bank, holding the mower on course by means of a length of rope tied to the machine. This takes the strain off the operator and is good assurance of a happy ending. If you have a riding mower, use it with extreme caution on steep inclines; it can tip over easily.

Particularly shocking and senseless are the many serious accidents among young children not involved in the mowing job. In Royal Oak, Mich., a father left the mower running while he went to the garage; his five-year-old son mangled his foot badly when he stuck it in the machine. In West Plains, Mo., a four-year-old boy had his leg broken and gashed to the bone while his fatner was oiling the running motor. *Never, never leave a mower running unattended for any reason.* Keep children (and pets) at a safe distance while you are working. Never let a child play with the mower any more than you would allow him to play with a loaded revolver. Power mowers—like other power tools, like guns and automobiles—are safe only when handled with full understanding of their dangers.

Safety Guide for Mower Buyers

In shopping for a rotary mower, look for a machine that has:

- Built-in guards covering dangerous revolving parts.
- A handle that won't flip over the top of the mower in a sudden stop.
- A grass-ejection slot with a deflector to limit the distance objects picked up by the blade are thrown.
- A grounded three-prong plug for electric mowers.
- Large wheels to simplify operation over uneven ground.
- A rear shield to keep feet away from the blade and to deflect objects.
- The gas tank away from the exhaust. This helps prevent fire.
- A "dead-man" device, which disengages the blade from the mower's power source when the operator lets go of the handle. This lets a brake stop the blade quickly.
- Finally, *try it before you buy it*. Choose only a mower that will be easy to maneuver on your terrain, and not too heavy or awkward for your physique.

CHAPTER TWO

PROTECT
YOUR CHILDREN

Can't We Stop These Tragic Injuries to Children?

by George W. Starbuck, M.D.

As a PEDIATRICIAN, it is my daily privilege to witness the miracle of parental love—that outpouring of tender devotion that wells forth, especially when sickness threatens a child. But I am sure I speak for all physicians when I say that we are constantly appalled by the way so many otherwise wonderful parents fail to take the most obvious precautions to prevent accidents from striking down their children.

The case of Susie G. is typical. Before she was born, her mother pored over booklets about baby care. Later, her mother conscientiously brought her to my office for inoculations and followed my feeding instructions religiously. But when Susie was only 21 months old, her mother left her in the kitchen "for just a minute" to hang up washing outdoors. During that "minute" the little tyke climbed on a chair and started a handkerchief through the electric wringer. The result: three fingers badly crushed, one broken and a hand in splints for weeks.

Because pediatricians so often have to treat such cases, we know that accidents, today, are the greatest of all child-cripplers—even child-killers. We know, too, from years of research and repeated studies that *nine out of every ten of these accidents need never happen.* Prevention is at hand: simple, common-sense steps that require less effort than taking a child for a polio vaccination. Unfortunately, however, a tragic apathy keeps too many parents from applying them. Every year, according to estimates, children under 15 years of age suffer the shocking total of between 16,000,000 and 20,000,000 accidental injuries. Many millions of these accidents are severe enough to require a physician's attention.

Each year approximately 40,000 to 50,000 youngsters are permanently maimed and over 9,000 lose their lives in accidents which, almost without exception, could have been prevented.

For nearly four decades pediatricians have been conducting a drive to reduce this dreadful toll. Through the Committee on Accident Prevention of the American Academy of Pediatrics, we helped the paint-making industries devise low-lead and leadless paints for toys and other objects, to reduce the danger of lead poisoning among children. A campaign to eliminate highly flammable fabrics in children's clothing has resulted in a federal law prohibiting interstate commerce in these dangerous garments. Refrigerators are now so designed that children cannot accidentally lock themselves in, to be doomed to slow death by suffocation. Poison control centers have been set up in most states, providing physicians with instant identification of the poisonous ingredients in common household products and with directions for emergency treatment.

Through these efforts, thousands of lives have already been saved. But we have made all too little progress in eliminating the greatest cause of childhood accidents: the parents' fatalistic belief that accidents are bound to happen. The truth is that a whole chain of events precedes every injury suffered by a child, and every time we fail to break that chain—by not removing a hazard, or by not teaching a child to avoid a danger—we help an accident to happen. It is essential that parents and other members of the family learn how to prevent accidents to children.

Infants, of course, need absolute protection. They must never be left alone on anything from which they may fall. Abandoned in a bathinette, even for the moment it takes to answer an insistent phone, they can roll over and drown. Unless their crib bars are closely spaced, they can wedge their heads between them. They can smother in pillows or blankets. Since they will suck any handy object, never refinish nursery furniture or toys with paint containing lead. Nor should we let them handle any small objects lest they pop them into their mouths and choke. Over 1000 babies are killed each year by accidents, most of which occur because someone failed to take seemingly "obvious" safety measures.

As soon as a child begins to toddle, he will need protection against an ever-growing number of hazards. In my home town of New Bedford, Mass., accident studies showed that 39 percent of all injuries to children are the result of falls. A tremendous proportion of these occur because parents fail to use a safety belt on the bathinette, or safety gates at the top and bottom of stairs or on porches.

Twenty-nine percent of childhood accidents in New Bedford were reported to have been caused by blows of one sort or another. Parents leave closet doors open, for instance, and youngsters, with their normal curiosity, reach to high shelves and pull down upon their heads all sorts of objects, from sharp-edged canisters to heavy electric irons. Twelve percent of our New Bedford accidents involved piercing injuries—the result of letting active children run around with pointed scissors and sharp-edged toys.

These are just a few examples of the scores of hazards that endanger children in every home. The only sure way to remove major hazards in *your* home is to list them one by one—and then eliminate them. Nor will it be enough to make such a list once. For, as your child learns to roam and explore, things that weren't a danger at first will quickly become acute menaces.

The kitchen is the most fascinating room to children—and the most dangerous. One study of accidents has revealed that about 15 percent of all fatal home accidents occur there. Children used to learn quickly to stay away from a coal stove or to keep their hands out of the clearly visible gas flames. But electric stoves are booby traps for youngsters unless we keep them from putting their fingers on surfaces they cannot know are hot. Common sense should tell us—but too often doesn't— to buy stoves with switches that children cannot reach and to keep pot handles turned so that toddlers can't grasp them and bring scalding food down on their heads.

Food mixers, dishwashers, can openers, garbage-disposal units are deadly threats to little children unless we arrange our homes so that they cannot get at them. So, too, are the products that cram our kitchen and laundry shelves. Medicine cabinets, once considered the prime source of danger from poisoning, are dangerous enough; but over 20 percent of the thousands of child poisonings that occur every year are caused by products thoughtlessly left in the kitchen where children can reach them: detergents, water softeners, waxes, furniture polishes, insecticides, etc.

On our lawns and in our yards, hundreds of youngsters have been injured by stones and wires hurled by rotary mowers from a distance of 10, 15, even 20 feet. Electric hedge clippers, saws, axes, etc., are all too attractive to tots if not stored out of reach, and they can inflict terrible slashes in an instant. The pesticides we store in our garages are a constant invitation to death if we don't keep them under lock and key.

Our cars—we should think of them as a mobile part of our homes— are another prime source of childhood accidents. Research has proved that the safest place, by all odds, is in the rear seat. Yet, millions of us will carry a baby on our laps in the front seat, beside the driver, the No. 1 danger spot in case of a sudden stop or a collision. Or we will leave a child in a parked car while we dash out to do a moment's shopping. (It takes only a minute for him to open a window or door and fall out, or to release the brake and roll off to disaster.) As adults, we can weigh the risks when we decide whether or not to use safety belts ourselves. But when we deny such belts—or an inexpensive safety seat with a strap—to our children, we are abetting an accident.

No matter how much forethought you apply, it is impossible to make a house *completely* accident-proof. Hence the conscientious parent never ceases to enforce rules about avoidable dangers in the child's environment. Above all, be consistent. If you forbid your child to handle scissors or matches or knives, never get teased into saying, "Okay— just this once." Perhaps the most important thing to remember is that young children find security in having clear limits set as to what they may do and may not do—as long as you couple your orders with praise for accomplishment and with permission to try some new things.

We pediatricians have found that parents who fail to teach their children how to protect themselves are the ones whose youngsters turn up most frequently in our offices and hospital emergency rooms. Time and again we have found that parents who enforce sensible precautions against injury—calmly, consistently, repeatedly—bring their children through the formative years with a minimum of bumps, scrapes and broken limbs. And when the youngsters go out into the world of schools, streets, playgrounds, beaches, and swimming pools, they carry with them ingrained habits of safety that will protect them even when parents cannot watch over them.

When Children Are In The Car

by Ken W. Purdy

THE CAR was a new station wagon, the driver a woman of 32, the passenger her three-year-old son standing upright in the front seat. The place was a shopping center in a small Connecticut town. The car was moving no faster than ten m.p.h. when a dog popped out in front of it. The driver hit the brake pedal—and the child was tossed at the dashboard like a rag doll. He wasn't badly hurt: a three-stitch cut in the right side of his forehead. His mother, the driver, was furious at the woman who had unleashed her dog. She would really have been outraged had she been told, as she should have been, that *she* had almost killed her own son.

The value of the auto seat belt has been established beyond question: seat belts reduce the chance of adult injury and death in auto accidents by at least 60 percent. The statistics on children are harder to come by, but thousands of children are injured every year, many in low-speed, unreported accidents like the one above. If you're driving at 15 m.p.h. and stop the car instantly, either by hitting the brakes or by running into something, everything in your car that isn't fastened down will continue to move forward at 15 m.p.h. until something stops it. Think of it this way: the metal dashboard of an automobile, swung 15 m.p.h. at the head of a 265-pound pro football player, can kill *him*, never mind a three-year-old child.

Adult seat belts are not suitable for very small children. For them, specially designed seating restraints are available on the market. Nine states now have laws requiring seating restraints for small children. Still, we see parents blithely driving along with children standing up.

The safest American driver, according to a study by the California Department of Motor Vehicles, is the married woman over 25. There are, I believe, reasons for this: often her driving is short-haul, low-speed; her accidents are frequently the short-stop, side-scrape, fender-bender kind, not serious enough to report, and so not included in the statistical record.

Are all of these women *really* good drivers? I don't think so. Some only *appear* to be good. One of the worst I know is a 43-year-old mother of five who has never had a traffic ticket or a reportable accident; statistically she's a superior driver, but actually she's terrible. She parks by moving the car until she feels the bumper hit something solid. She would be helpless in an emergency. She's indifferent to the maintenance of the car—as long as it will run and she can see through the windshield, she's happy. I wouldn't ride five miles with her if I could help it.

Given the special circumstances in which parent-drivers operate, here are some tips that will help them to be better drivers:

• Some people tend to think of the automobile as just another household appliance. It is our most valuable convenience, but it's also a deadly device in which over 50,000 Americans a year die and 40 times that many suffer disabling injuries. Treat it with respect. When you step on the accelerator, you may be dealing with as much as 400 horsepower. Would you snap a whip over a herd of 400 actual horses?

• Don't drive a sick automobile. If it takes longer to stop than usual, if it pulls to one side when you're braking, if you can move the steering wheel a couple of inches before the car begins to turn—have it fixed immediately. The cost is small. Learn the routine facts of maintenance: how much air is supposed to be in the tires (very important for safety); how to tell if the engine needs oil; how to check the brake-fluid level (your life may depend on a couple of teacups of fluid). Get out at a gas station to make sure the attendant is making checks properly. I've seen one, talking to a friend while he worked, put 50 pounds of air into a tire rated at 24.

• Enforce a family rule: If the car is moving, everybody's seat belt is fastened. No exceptions.

• Confine children to the back seat if possible. Lock the doors. Don't carry sharp or heavy objects on the same seats with children. Don't put anything on the shelf under the back window. In a sudden stop even a camera, flying forward at the original speed of the car, can be lethal.

• Put the groceries in the trunk. In a station wagon, put them on the rear platform.

• Never leave small children alone in the car. If you leave children old enough to obey and remember, put the transmission in Park, put the brake on, and take the ignition key. If the car has power windows that will work with the ignition off, be certain that your children can be positively trusted not to play with them. Power windows have strangled small children.

• Everyone who must drive in snowy country should learn how to handle a skid—actually practice skidding, on a driving-school or police skidpan if possible, or on a deserted parking lot or a wide driveway. If, instinctively, you put on the brakes in a skid, you'll make the skid much worse. Basically, you must take your foot off the gas and turn in the direction that you want the front end of the car to go. You can't learn without trying it.

• The only safe driver is one who anticipates, and so almost never gets into a situation requiring violent braking or acceleration. In an emergency, there is no time to think: an accident can be all over in .8 second; an emergency lasting two seconds is a long one. So memorize some emergency decisions. For example:

If swerving to avoid hitting an animal will throw you into an oncoming car, hit the animal.

A ball rolling in the street means a child chasing it. Slow to a crawl.

If you hear tire squeal, you're doing something wrong: accelerating too hard, braking too hard, going too fast in a curve.

In passing situations, a car coming straight at you looks much the same doing 100 m.p.h. as it does doing 30. When in doubt, don't pass. When you *do* pass, don't dawdle—get it over with, but do it safely.

If Junior is beating up his sister in the back seat, don't look in the mirror, and don't turn around. Stop the car off the road.

Light rain after a dry spell means a road slippery as glass. (Rain mixes with oil film and dirt.) Slow down, increase the distance between you and other cars, drive with extra alertness.

At night, when an approaching driver leaves his brights on, don't get even by turning yours on. Why should *both* of you be blind?

In normal weather conditions the safest speed is the speed of the traffic stream you're driving in.

Try to come up with some emergency rules of your own. Driving is a serious business, and anything that makes you think about it helps make you safer behind the wheel.

CHAPTER THREE

POISON:
HANDLE WITH CARE

Home Canning:
The Safe Way

by Jean Carper

FROM APARTMENT DWELLERS to farmers' wives, from community groups to family gardeners, a record-breaking 19 to 23 million Americans canned foods at home in 1976. Home canning was once the exclusive purview of the housewife, but men and young people are now taking it up, too. Why the boom?

Many feel their own canned foods are purer and taste better. For others, it's an esthetic pleasure combined with nostalgia. "Canning for us is a family affair where we all pitch in," says a Washington, D.C., mother. "We love the smells of the jellies boiling in the kitchen and the bright colors of the jars all lined up on the shelves." Canning can also be a way of saving money, in spite of the initial investment in equipment.

Home canning is an essentially simple method of using heat to *sterilize* the jar and its food contents, killing all spoilage- and disease-producing micro-organisms. Unfortunately, a lot of people—even long-time canners—are doing it wrong. Canning methods have changed, and what you learned from your mother or even from canning manuals five years ago may no longer be valid.

Essentially, only two things can go wrong: food can spoil or be contaminated with the deadly toxin that causes botulism. During canning, the thousands of different kinds of bacteria, yeasts and molds that are in the air, on jars and in the food itself must be killed by heat. And then the jar must be tightly sealed to prevent new contamination. How much heat depends on many factors, including the type of bacteria or other micro-organisms, plus the acidity and density of food being canned.

One of the most heat-resistant bacteria is *Clostridium botulinum* in its spore form, which can thrive in improperly canned low-acid foods such as fish and green beans. If a single botulinum spore survives in a jar, within a short time under suitable conditions it will give rise to 500 million botulinum cells, all producing potentially deadly toxin. Eating only one spoonful of botulinum-contaminated food can be fatal.

But there's no need to fear these hazards—if you do your canning properly. Here are some important tips which will help you ensure home-canning success:

1. *Get reliable instructions.* Amazingly, many home canners have never so much as glanced at an instruction booklet. The most dependable information comes from the U.S. Department of Agriculture (USDA) and is often reprinted in other booklets. Some major canning-equipment manufacturers also publish helpful information.

2. *Follow instructions exactly.* If they say to leave ½-inch space at the top of the jar, don't leave ¾ inch; if they say the food should be processed in a pressure canner for 25 minutes, that doesn't mean 22 minutes. There is good scientific reason behind the precision of the instructions.

   You can also get in trouble by altering recipes. Adding thickening agents, for example, retards heat penetration, throwing off processing timetables. If you're going to use cherries for pie filling, or beef and vegetables for stew, thicken them at the time of use, not before canning. And if you mix vegetables such as carrots, green beans, lima beans and celery, use the maximum processing time required for any single vegetable in your combination. The best advice is: don't make up your own recipes.

3. *Avoid the open-kettle method for all foods but jellies.* This system

of heating the food to boiling in an open kettle and then putting it in jars is a common practice that leads to spoilage. Even if jars are sterilized, transferring food from the kettle exposes it to yeasts, molds and bacteria in the air. Moreover, the contaminants can be sealed in the jar and may continue to grow.

4. *Use a boiling-water bath for all acid foods*—pickled vegetables, relishes, sauerkraut and fruits, including those in jams, marmalades, preserves. In this method, the properly filled and closed jars are submerged in hot or boiling water in a covered container with a rack, and boiled for the prescribed time to kill all spoilage micro-organisms. Be sure the boiling water is an inch or two over the tops of the jars the entire time—add more boiling water if necessary—and start timing *after* the water is at full boil. If directions call for 15 minutes or less in the water bath, it's best to sterilize jars before packing with food.

5. *Use a pressure canner for low-acid foods.* Nothing is more crucial in preventing botulism in canning vegetables, meats, poultry, fish and every other food not specifically designated high acid. Some canners mistakenly think a pressure canner is recommended because it is quicker and that instead they can simply increase the heating time in the boiling-water-bath method to get the same results. This is not so. Water baths never get above 212 degrees F., the boiling point of water. It is the *pressure* in the canner that brings the temperature to the 240 degrees F. necessary to kill botulinum spores. Be sure the pressure is at the prescribed level— usually ten or fifteen pounds—before you start timing and keep the pressure at that point by adjusting the burner.

If you are buying a new pressure canner, choose one made by a reputable manufacturer. You can get good medium- and large-size pressure canners for about $45 to $90 and smaller ones for about $30 to $45.

Pressure canners come with either dial pressure or weighted gauge. The latter doesn't get out of kilter, but the former can, giving you an inaccurate reading. Have the dial checked before every canning season or more often if used frequently. Your county extension agent or local dealer can probably tell you where this service is available.

6. *Don't use "shortcuts."* Aspirin, boric acid or other so-called preservatives do not prevent spoilage. That's all folklore. The correct heat treatment is the only safe procedure to use in home canning. Although it may seem logical that setting jars of food in a 450-degree F. oven would do the job, studies show the internal temperature in such jars does not go above boiling, which is not high enough to kill botulinum spores. Jars are also apt to break or explode in the oven. Because of its fluctuating temperature and dry heat, the oven should never be used for canning.

7. *Pay special attention to tomatoes.* Because of their high-acid content, tomatoes have long been regarded as free of the botulism hazard. Some experts still say it's all right to use the boiling-water bath. However, through the years, a few new tomato varieties have been developed which are less acid, and the foolproof protection is now evidently gone.

As a safeguard, other experts suggest adding acid. For each quart of tomatoes mix in 1/2 teaspoon of citric acid (available at most drugstores). Or use two teaspoons of canned or bottled lemon juice or two teaspoons of five-percent vinegar. Don't use fresh lemon juice; lemons, too, have become less acid through the years and can't be relied on. Do not use tomatoes that are overripe or unsound. These may have too little acid for canning.

8. *Use proper jars and lids.* Don't use old mayonnaise, peanut butter, or any other so-called "one-trip" jars from the supermarket. These are usually not the exact size and shape needed to accommodate standard canning lids. The glass may also break at high temperatures. Some canners are turning to antique jars, but these may have hairline cracks, causing them to break when heated.

Be alert: some ill-designed lids are on the market. Stick to those you know, and never buy lids that are not explicitly labeled for canning or that fail to include both directions for use and the name and address of the manufacturer. It's best to stay with the same manufacturer year after year. The sealing compound of lids varies from manufacturer to manufacturer, and you learn from experience how much pressure to apply when sealing a jar with a particular type of lid.

9. *Be sure of a good seal.* Besides killing micro-organisms, the purpose of heat in canning is to drive air out of the jar to form a vacuum seal. If you don't get a seal, or if it breaks after several days, probable reasons are: wrong-type or damaged jar or lid, screwband not sufficiently tightened (but do not tighten screwbands or zinc lids *after* processing unless the manufacturer so specifies or you may break the seal), incorrect processing, food or grease lodged between the lid and jar. The last happens if you fill the jar too full, fail to wipe off the mouth before applying lid or pack foods raw.

How can you tell if you get a good seal? As a test, after 12 to 24 hours, lightly press the flat lid; if it is down and won't move, it is sealed. With zinc porcelain-lined lids, tip the jar slightly to be sure no liquid seeps out. If the jar isn't sealed, use the food immediately or can it again.

10. *Be careful with hot foods.* If you are canning cooked food, do not let it cool. Fill the jars and begin processing immediately. Don't pack hot food too tightly, or you won't have the heat penetration required.

If you do everything right, you shouldn't have more than one out of every 100,000 jars spoil. However, if you note any sign of spoilage—foam, off-odor, spurting liquid, bulging lid—don't taste the food. Throw it out. Foods that contain the toxin that causes botulism may show no signs of spoilage. So it's best never to taste a home-canned, low-acid food before boiling it at least ten minutes and even longer for denser foods such as meat, seafood or corn.

Moldy jams and jellies were once thought safe if you scraped off the mold, but some evidence indicates that mold grows down in invisible threads, in some cases adversely affecting the contents. And some molds produce toxins which can be health hazards. To be safe, discard moldy home-canned food.

Does home canning save money? A 1978 study showed that if you had the jars and got tomatoes or green beans free, for example, you could put them up for about four cents a quart. The same study indicated that if you had to buy produce and jars, a quart might have cost 60 cents for tomatoes and 56 cents for green beans, compared with 78 to 95 cents and 74 to 98 cents, respectively, for a national brand in the supermarket. So it may be cheaper to can. Beyond that, it gives millions of gardeners the chance to enjoy their produce for months after it has been harvested.

Tips on Freezing

Freezing fresh food is more expensive than canning because of electrical costs, but some people prefer the texture and taste of frozen foods. Here are some general rules for freezing.

- Use moisture-proof and vapor-proof containers designed especially for freezing; other containers will let food dry out, causing "freezer-burn" and loss of flavor, color and texture.
- Blanch practically all vegetables before freezing, following directions from the USDA or other reputable sources. Without such heat treatment, the enzymes in vegetables cause them to continue to "ripen" even though frozen, making them discolored and tough, and changing their taste.
- Get as much air as possible out of containers by packing food tightly or squeezing air out of bags after they're packed. Then seal firmly before freezing. Air trapped in containers causes freezer burn. However, allow some space; food expands when frozen and if packed too tightly, may rupture the container.
- Freeze food quickly so it doesn't lose quality or spoil. Don't put more unfrozen food in the freezer than will freeze within 24 hours—usually two to three pounds per cubic foot of freezer—and leave a little space between containers so air can circulate freely. Once food is frozen, store containers close together.
- Always keep food frozen at 0 degrees F. or below. At higher temperatures food will lose quality.

Food Poisoning— And How to Avoid It

by James H. Winchester

SIX CLOSE relatives gathered at the home of Mr. and Mrs. Dan Hughes one June evening to celebrate a family birthday. For dinner they had fried chicken with gravy, canned corn, salad, mashed potatoes, beans and cake. Before midnight, the visiting kin said good-by.

Shortly after 1 a.m., the happy occasion began to develop into a nightmare. Mrs. Hughes awakened with a splitting headache, stomach cramps and diarrhea. Her husband was just as ill, and before morning the Hughes children were also doubled up with pain, as was their grandmother. Before the day was over, everyone present at the party had been hospitalized. All were suffering from food poisoning.

One of the most common causes of illness in the world, food poisoning, hits well over a million Americans each year. It occurs in a variety of ways. Bacteria overrun foods, attacking stomach and intestinal tissues directly or creating a toxin that is just as inflammatory. Chemicals from sprays and fertilizers often contaminate foods.

In the Hughes case, laboratory analysis showed that a bacterium known as Salmonella had done the dirty work.

Salmonellosis produces cramps, nausea, headache, vomiting, prostration, severe diarrhea and dehydration. More than 20,000 cases were reported in 1964. In investigating for causes, researchers in Cincinnati discovered that one out of every six chickens picked up on the open

45

market there carried Salmonella germs; other tests of nationwide samples have revealed that as much as 36 percent of fryer chickens, 12 percent of fresh pork sausage and one percent of ground beef may be similarly contaminated.

Nothing much can be done for sufferers except to prescribe fluids and sometimes bed rest. Healthy persons throw off the infection themselves, usually within three to five days. Babies and persons weakened by other ailments, however, often can't cope with the disease. In 1963, 601 hospital patients came down with salmonellosis, and 16 died. "It's the nation's No. 1 food-poisoning problem," reports Dr. Philip S. Brachman, chief of the epidemiology program office at the Centers for Disease Control in Atlanta, Ga.

Investigating at the Hughes home, health officials found large numbers of *Salmonella newport*, one of the more than 1500 known strains of the germ, in the leftover chicken and gravy. Careful questioning revealed what had happened. Eight chickens, raised in the Hughes backyard, had been killed two weeks earlier, then dressed and frozen immediately. Early on the morning of the party, they were taken from the freezer and put in open pans in the kitchen to thaw. At 3 p.m. they were quick-fried; then they were put on the back of the stove until dinnertime.

The Salmonella were thought to have been present in the chickens when they were killed. (Health officials suspect that germs in raw-meat scraps and fish meal that go into animal feeds are a possible source of infection.) Freezing curbs but does not kill these germs. During the thaw-out in the Hughes kitchen the germs revived and propagated, and the cooking was neither hot enough nor long enough to kill them. Only *very thorough* cooking kills Salmonella in meats. County health authorities could do nothing but warn the Hughes family to be more careful in the future.

Less acute than salmonellosis, but more common, are staphylococcus infections carried by food. Staphylococcus germs in themselves are not harmful to the digestive tract; but in food they can produce an extremely irritating toxin which causes symptoms somewhat similar to those of salmonellosis (but shorter-lasting—generally less than a day). Carelessness on the part of the food handler is frequently a cause. Everyone at some time or other carries staphylococcus germs around in nose and throat, or on the skin. Unsanitary utensils may be loaded with them. Cured meats, sandwich preparations, salads (particularly tuna-fish, chicken, potato), milk and cream-filled bakery goods are excellent spawning grounds for staph bacteria.

When a southern businessman entertained friends at a backyard picnic, his wife cooked a ham for the occasion. She sneezed several times while preparing the meat, apparently infecting the ham and the knife she was using. Though the cooking killed the germs in the meat, the knife was not washed before being used to slice the ham, and the meat became reinfected. In the summer heat, the germs doubled themselves about twice an hour, and everyone who ate the ham fell ill. Health investigators found later that portions of the sliced ham yielded nearly five billion staph germs per gram.

While salmonellosis and staphylococcus infections are the most prevalent food diseases, botulism is the most dangerous. It can cause respiratory failure and death. Botulism spores are harmless in themselves; everyone swallows many of them daily on raw fruits and vegetables. But in a warm, airless environment such as that of a hermetically sealed can, they sometimes produce a deadly toxin which attacks the central nervous system 12 to 36 hours after a contaminated food has been eaten. One hundred-billionth of a gram of pure botulism toxin is lethal to a mouse when injected; cobra venom is mild by comparison.

Most outbreaks of botulism in the United States in this century have been traced to home canning, generally resulting from failure to cook the food at temperatures high enough and long enough (240°–250° F. for 15 to 90 minutes, depending on the product and the size of the can) to kill the botulism spores. Low-acid foods are usually involved. String beans seem to have a particular affinity, as do corn, beets, asparagus, pork products, seafood, spinach, peppers, figs and mushrooms.

Though the disease is relatively rare—only 1561 cases were reported in the United States from 1899 through 1963—14 persons died of it in 1963. Nine of these fatalities, and more than half of all the cases, stemmed from commercially processed foods. In Michigan, two women died after eating tainted canned tuna fish. In Tennessee, smoked white-fish, which had been shipped from the Great Lakes in an unrefrigerated truck, was responsible for several other deaths. As a result, improved methods of smoking, freezing, packaging and shipping fish are now being enforced by the U.S. Food and Drug Administration.

Still a formidable health threat, too, is trichinosis, which comes from eating undercooked pork. Tiny worms from the infected meat are released in the intestinal tract and carried by the bloodstream to muscle tissues, where they cause swelling, muscular pain and diarrhea. The muscular weakness may be prolonged and disabling, and in some cases death results.

Cases decreased in the early 1960s because of state and local laws forbidding the feeding of raw garbage to hogs. But serious outbreaks still occur, and autopsy studies in 1970 indicated that about two percent of the U.S. population may be infected with the disease.

How can you protect yourself and your family against food poisoning? Here are the precautions advised by the Public Health Service:

• Always wash your hands before preparing food.

• For picnics, take along as many non-perishable foods as possible, such as potato chips and well-scrubbed raw fruits and vegetables. Use a portable cooler for salads and perishable items. Barbecuing on the spot is a good idea—if the food is eaten while still hot.

• Food prepared in advance, as well as leftovers, should be refrigerated immediately and never left standing.

• Salad dressings, éclairs, cream puffs and custard-type desserts should be kept refrigerated until just before serving. Otherwise they become excellent mediums for germ incubation.

• Keep hot foods hot and cold foods cold, either at more than 140° F. or at less than 40° F. Avoid letting food sit at in-between, lukewarm temperatures at which bacteria thrive.

"Help!
My Child
Has Taken Poison!"

by Evan McLeod Wylie

Accidental poisoning is one of the most common emergencies in child-hood. Every year about a million poison cases involving U.S. children are reported, and hundreds of these children die. Thanks to the efforts of the public-health and medical professions, more than 500 poison-control centers now stand ready to give parents, patients, doctors and hospitals immediate information about what to do in all poisoning emergencies. This dramatic report is drawn from the author's first-hand observations at one of the nation's busiest centers.

TELEPHONES were ringing in all three rooms of a suite on the third floor of the huge downtown building that serves as headquarters for the New York City Department of Health. The brightly illuminated rooms were cluttered with battered desks, filing cabinets, and bookcases crammed with volumes bearing such titles as *Dangerous Properties of Industrial Materials, Accidental Poisoning in Childhood,* and *Clinical Toxicology of Commercial Products.* Three men—Jim Grennan, Milton Goldberg and Harry Raybin—were talking on phones, jotting down notes, and searching through books and stacks of file folders.

Raybin punched a button on a ringing phone and said, "This is Poison Control." An excited young woman said, "I need help fast! I can't get my doctor. My two-year-old son swallowed laundry bleach!"

"Now, take it easy," Raybin said. "Read me the label." His voice was soft but alert. "Do you know how much of it he took?"

"The container was about three-quarters empty," the woman said.

"Then, since the label said 12 fluid ounces, the most your boy could have taken was around three ounces," Raybin reassured her. "I can tell you right now that it won't hurt him. Just give him a good drink of milk. That will help neutralize the chemicals of that particular bleach."

Though it was nearing dinner time on the Atlantic seaboard, the New York Poison Control Center gave no sign of closing shop. It never does: the center operates 24 hours a day the year round, and its phones seldom stop ringing. It works closely with 170 hospitals in the East Coast region and regularly receives emergency calls from hospitals, doctors, other poison-control centers as far away as California, Hawaii and Canada, and from ships at sea. When Harry Raybin, a chemist specializing in toxicology, and the center's director, goes home in the evening, he is still accessible to the staff on duty. "If we get into a tight situation, we call him," Grennan says. "He's got more information in his head than you'd find in any of these files."

Grennan took the next call. A nurse from the Central Valley Hospital in New Jersey was reporting the case of three-year-old Tommy Gibson. His mother had been preparing for a cookout. She had momentarily left her son alone on the patio. Tommy had picked up the can of charcoal lighter fluid and drunk it. Mrs. Gibson had called her doctor, who instructed her to take Tommy to the hospital at once.

"Any vomiting or choking?" Grennan asked.

"None."

"Can you tell me the brand name?" Grennan asked. "Did the mother bring in the container?"

"Let me check," the nurse said.

"Knowing the brand in these cases can help us a lot," Raybin explained to me. "There are two kinds of charcoal lighter fluid. One is a wood alcohol. The other, a mixture of petroleum products, particularly kerosene, is a bad actor. If even a small amount is sucked into the lungs when the child chokes or vomits, there's a real hazard to his life."

Now the nurse was back on Grennan's phone. "The mother forgot to bring the container, but her husband is on his way here. We'll get the name from him."

Grennan warned the nurse not to attempt a gastric lavage (stomach washing) or use an emetic, because of the risk in gagging and vomiting. "We normally recommend close observation for signs of chemical pneumonia in case the child choked on the material and got it in his lungs."

In child poisoning, Harry Raybin said between calls, the peak danger age is three. The two- and three-year-olds are immensely curious. They're exploring, putting everything in their mouths. They're climbers. The one-year-olds are the creepers. They get the stuff near the floor—under the kitchen sink, in the utility room—detergents, furniture polish, cleaning solvents, bleaches. The older ones get the pills, medicines and outdoor poisons.

"You'd be surprised where the child finds the medicines," Raybin said. "People used to keep them in the medicine chest. Now they're all over the place. Women leave sugar-coated iron pills on the dining-room table. Tranquilizers and birth-control pills, too."

Every parent should keep in mind, Raybin said, that most child poisonings occur between noon and 6 p.m. when small children are active and the home is the busiest. The mother or father is preoccupied, working or talking on the telephone—then suddenly the baby's got a mouthful of something!

"Any time a child is left alone is dangerous," Raybin added. "On Sunday morning, for example, when the parents sleep late and the little ones are roaming around. That's when we get a lot of our 'baby-aspirin' poisonings. Aspirin causes over six percent of all poison fatalities in children. You know, there are plenty of parents who still describe aspirin to children as 'candy.'"

"Is there an antidote for it?" I asked.

"No," Raybin replied. "There's a popular belief that there is a specific antidote for most poisons. That just isn't so. We have files of information about dangerous chemicals and drugs, and reports by drug companies and the National Clearinghouse for Poison Control Centers in Rockville, Md., but usually the best we can come up with is the proper course of emergency treatment. For aspirin, we try to get the stuff up—make them vomit. But in some poison cases, that's the worst thing to do. It may only cause more damage to the esophagus or introduce the poison into the lungs.

"Our job is to find out exactly what happened, quickly analyze the problem, suggest treatment, and warn about side effects and after effects. Often the best answer is immediate dilution of the poison—with the appropriate fluid—and then rapid elimination before the toxic substance is absorbed."

"Poison Control," said Goldberg, taking the next call.

"This is Dr. Taylor at the Hospital for Crippled Children," a voice said. "I have a two-year-old girl who has taken camphorated oil."

"How much, doctor?" Goldberg asked.

"About three teaspoonfuls."

"You ought to get it out of her right away," Goldberg said. "It's very toxic." He cautioned the doctor about the possibility of convulsions, and recommended washing out the child's stomach.

"Camphor creates a lot of problems," Raybin commented. "It's in mothballs, ointments, flakes and in the medicinal oil. It can make a child awfully sick—even kill him."

Grennan took another call: a nurse in a Connecticut hospital, saying, "A 16-month-old child has taken a white liquid. Her lips are burned and she's screaming." The container, the nurse said, was a plain, unlabeled bottle.

"Where did she get it? What part of her house?"

"In the basement. They found her crying beside the bottle."

Grennan frowned. "It could be lye. Do a pH test right away. And I think you ought to get some water into her. Then call us back."

As he waited, he said, "Kids still get their hands on lye. It's one of the worst because it burns and scars the esophagus so they have to have surgery later."

He took the return call from the hospital. The pH test showed an acid reaction.

"Then it can't be lye," Grennan said. "Did you give her the water?"

"She doesn't want to take anything," the nurse said.

"Squeeze her cheeks together gently with your fingers until she opens her mouth, then pour in a little at a time," Grennan said. "She's bound to swallow some. It will help dilute that stuff she took. Then follow up by having an eye, ears, nose and throat specialist look into her mouth and down her throat to see if there are any burns. If there are, you'll need to take certain precautions, and she'll require special treatment. If there are other problems, call us back."

He replaced the receiver. "It makes you sore," he said, "when you think of the way people leave all kinds of 'hot stuff' in bottles—lye, paint thinners, solvents, rat poison. Often it's in a soda-pop bottle that a kid is naturally going to take a drink from. Most child poisonings are due to some adult's carelessness."

Now the nurse from Central Valley Hospital called back about Tommy Gibson. She gave Jim Grennan the name of the charcoal lighter fluid. Grennan sighed into the phone. "That's a petroleum product. But no symptoms so far? Well, tonight will tell the story. Close observation is important."

"We're sending him home with his mother," the nurse said. "But we have instructed her to take his temperature every two hours."

"Absolutely," Grennan said. "If he got lighter fluid in his lungs, there will be temperature and lung complications. You will want to yank him back in fast."

Goldberg put a pot of coffee on a hot plate to percolate. The men now took a flurry of calls, shuttling back and forth between phones and files, flipping through books and folders.

A father reported that his two-year-old son had swallowed half a bottle of nose drops; a Pennsylvania mother said that her one-year-old had bitten into a tube of nail-beauty cream. Then a doctor called: a 45-year-old woman had taken an overdose of sleeping pills.

Goldberg, covering the mouthpiece, called to Grennan: "Suicide attempt—Nembutal." Grennan leaped up, yanked open a cabinet, pulled out a folder that included the manufacturer's report on overdosage, and put it in front of Goldberg.

"Can we dialyze her?" asked the doctor. (Dialysis means pumping the patient's blood through an artificial kidney to remove poisons.) "Yes," said Goldberg. He reeled off a list of hospitals with emergency dialysis equipment.

In the western sky a flicker of lightning and the rumble of thunder signaled an approaching storm. Jim Grennan got up to shut a window. "So far tonight," he said, "no fatalities. We're lucky. The only sure thing you can say about most child poisonings is that they didn't have to happen. And the best answer to the problem is one that would nearly put this place out of business: *prevention*."

Postscript:
Home Treatment
for Poisoning

A "Poison Safeguard Kit," manufactured by Marshall Electronics of Skokie, Ill., has now hit the consumer market. Approved by the non-profit National Poison Center Network, the kit contains two half-ounce bottles of syrup of ipecac for inducing vomiting, 25 grams of activated charcoal for absorbing poison, a bag for vomit, information on poison prevention and an instruction booklet written by Dr. Richard W. Moriarty, director of the 55-unit poison-center network. The booklet advises: "Call your poison center, a hospital emergency room or doctor first. *Do not* give the victim anything in this kit until told to do so."

Home treatment is adequate for 80 to 85 percent of an estimated five million poisonings in the United States each year, says Dr. Moriarty, an associate professor of pediatrics at the University of Pittsburgh. But usually people don't have on hand the proper drugs in the proper amounts. People could put their own kits together for considerably less than the $7.95 being asked—but, he notes, they rarely do.

—*Medical World News*

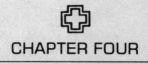

CHAPTER FOUR

HOUSE FIRE!

Is Your Home a Family Firetrap?

by Warren R. Young

WHEN Mary and Roger Wright took a ten-day vacation, they left their four children, ages four to eight, in the charge of a trusted elderly baby-sitter. Since the sitter had not previously stayed in their rambling, three-story house, Mrs. Wright left lengthy instructions—including mention of the children's fascination with some candles they had made at school, and her rule that they might light them only at mealtimes.

On the tenth morning, with the Wrights due home within hours, one child apparently began experimenting with a candle in a first-floor closet while the sitter was momentarily busy with the laundry. Returning from the basement, she saw flames in the living room. Scuttling back and forth to the kitchen, she tossed some water on the fire—with no effect. Seeing one child, she told him to get out; he and another child ran to a neighbor's house. Then she phoned the fire department.

Now she began looking for the other children. It was already too late. As she tried to go upstairs, heat singed her hair. Then smoke drove her outside. When the fire was brought under control, the seven-year-old boy and four-year-old girl were found dead from the hot toxic fumes on the third floor, where they had fled.

What makes this tragedy of the Wrights especially significant is that it was so similar in several key ways to many other fires in homes: the strange fascination that matches seem to hold for children; the uncertainty about what to do first—which always should be to *try to get everybody out*, even before phoning the fire department; the futility of fighting any but the tiniest fire by oneself; the shocking swiftness with which smoke, heat and fumes can build to killing levels even in rooms far from the actual flames.

Appallingly, every 45 seconds a fire breaks out in an American home—700,000 residences aflame each year. And 16 times a day somebody dies in one of these burning homes. More than 5800 people were killed this way in the United States in 1980.

Yet experts insist that nearly all these deaths are preventable. Robert W. Grant, president of the National Fire Protection Association, says, "If every family would take a few simple precautions, most of the people who now die in residential fires could escape alive." Analyses that the NFPA has made point to these six key steps to safeguard your family:

1. *Set strict smoking rules*. Careless handling of cigarettes, matches and other smoking materials sparks about one in every four fires in homes, and causes over 70 percent of all residential fire deaths. (Over one fourth of these fatalities result from smoking in bed, with even more caused by smoldering cigarettes falling into upholstered furniture.) If you don't want to ban smoking in your home (and today it is increasingly acceptable to forbid it), furnish large, non-tipping ashtrays. After smokers leave, check every sofa, chair, ashtray and wastebasket for unextinguished hazards. Allow nobody—family member or guest—to smoke in bed.

2. *Install smoke detectors*. Deadly fire gases, not flames themselves, cause three fourths of fire deaths in dwellings. Comparably high proportions of fatal fires begin as slow, smoldering affairs during the normal sleeping hours between 10 p.m. and 6 a.m., and involve a significant delay before anybody becomes aware of the burning.

The implications of such statistics have been clear to safety experts for years, but home fire-alarm systems generally reacted to heat alone. Only in the last decade has a moderately priced *smoke* detector been developed. Designs vary, but individual units, powered by household current or long-life batteries, that pick up the first abnormal whiffs of smoke and set off an alarm loud enough to rouse the deepest sleeper, can be bought for $10 to $25 each. You can install them yourself, and experts say that the average home would be far safer with detectors placed just outside the bedrooms. There should be one detector for each level of the house, including basement and attic.

3. *Sleep with bedroom doors closed.* This is the simplest safety precaution you can take, but it can be one of the most important. It is hard to realize, until an emergency comes, just how little time the toxic smoke and lethally hot air allow you for escape. A snug-fitting, solid-core wooden door, when shut, can treble the time it takes for a fire starting elsewhere to become intolerable or fatal inside your room.

4. *Have a family escape plan.* Not knowing what to do can make a person blunder into a deadly mistake. Teach members of your family what to expect before they ever confront a fire. Make them fully aware that, if a fire comes, it may be too dark to see (because of smoke or electrical failure); that breathing may be difficult and that normal exits may be blocked by heat and smoke. Everybody should know at least two ways out of every room, how to open windows and screens quickly, and how to use any folding ladders needed for upper windows. If your family includes infants, elderly persons, or handicapped persons, decide whose assignment it is to get them out.

Have periodic drills to give actual practice in the life-or-death rules. *First*, warn everybody. *Second*, get everybody out, fast. *Third*, get out yourself. *Fourth*, after everybody is out, call the fire department. (Know the nearest phone that can be reached outside your home.) Emphasize the urgency of swift action, without stopping to dress, gather belongings or fight the fire, unless it is still so small that it can be snuffed out in an instant. (For these situations, every home should have an approved fire extinguisher.)

Have everybody practice rising quickly from bed, going to the bedroom door, feeling it to see if it is hot or cool. (If hot, it must be left shut and another route taken; if cool, it may be opened, but warily lest a blast of superheated gas rush in.) Make clear that heat rises, hence the vital rule: "Stay low"—crawling can keep you below intolerable layers of hot toxic fumes. Your plan should include a meeting point, to prevent attempts to rescue persons already safe. Tell everybody: "Once out, stay out. Don't go back into a burning house, even to try a rescue."

5. *Keep a constant eye on the kids*. A disproportionate number of fire victims are children, and many of these victims are either alone or unsupervised at the time of the fire. Always keep matches and lighters beyond the reach of children (and remember that children are crafty explorers). When they are of school age, train them to handle matches carefully, with crystal-clear rules that they may light them only when you are with them. Teach them also to stay a safe distance from all open flames, cookstoves, sparks and hot electric coils.

6. *Inspect your home*. One reason that private houses turn into family firetraps more frequently than, say, hotels and apartment houses is that they are not given regular checkups for fire hazards. Use the following safety checklist.

Heating equipment.

Faulty heating equipment is the cause of more dwelling fires than smoking, and it is the runner-up to smoking in causing fatal residential fires. Has your furnace been inspected within a year? If you have gas-burning equipment, are you sure there are no leaks? Are flues, chimneys and fireplaces structurally sound and not coated with grease (from barbecues) or heavy layers of creosote? Are portable heaters (the most dangerous of all heating devices) in perfect condition, of approved design, fueled properly, and kept strictly away from combusitible materials?

Electrical equipment.

Does the wiring in your house have sufficient power-carrying capacity to all your appliances? The National Electrical Code now requires at least 100-amp service in a private dwelling, whereas in 1956 the approved standard was 60 amps. Thus, if your house was built before 1956, and has not had its electrical service modernized, you are probably in danger of overloading the wiring's capacity—and that could mean fire. (If you have any doubt, ask a qualified electrician to inspect your power panel.)

Make sure that if your house uses old-style, screw-in fuses, none of these are more than 15- or 20-amp capacity. Try not to use extension cords, especially on heat-producing appliances. If you must use them, make sure that every extension cord is in perfect condition, and bears the Underwriters Laboratories (UL) label showing that it meets safety standards. Double-check that none are wrapped around nails or hooks, tied in knots, run under rugs, strung through doorways, placed near a heat source or used for more than one appliance at a time.

Flammable material.

Is your stove kept free of greasy deposits? Are there oily rags or other sources of spontaneous combustion in your house? Are all paints, thinners, gasoline, adhesives, etc., in leakproof, tightly closed, shatterproof containers? They should be stored in a cool place, and those most easily ignited—such as gasoline—should be kept completely away from the house.

Family plan.

When you prepare your family's fire-escape plan, make certain that every escape route is clear of impediments. Will screens, storm windows and regular windows open easily? Do you have folding ladders and strong-beam, reliable flashlights where needed?

Review.

Does each family member know just what to do if fire strikes? Are the fire-department telephone number and your home address posted plainly beside every phone? Have all family members memorized that number?

REMEMBER: With just a little thought and preparation, these rules and safeguards can give you one of the best life-insuring plans possible.

ESDs—
Those Astonishing
Little Fire Alarms

by Edward Fales

ELECTRONIC SMOKE DETECTORS, remarkable little gadgets initially developed for industry and the military, are now on the retail market in large numbers. Experts acclaim them as far and away the best fire protection families have ever been offered. They're proving such effective lifesavers that twenty-five states now require them by law in all new houses, apartments and mobile homes. Eighteen other states have adopted requirements for existing housing. Some insurance companies even offer small rebates for their use.

Costing from $10 to $25, the detectors—called ESDs—are mounted up near or on the ceiling, where smoke goes first. Most run on batteries or have "plug-in" electric cords, and can be installed in moments with a screwdriver. Others are wired into house circuits. All contain horns or buzzers that sound an ear-piercing alarm; most reset automatically when the smoke clears. Often they are able to sense fire long before you can, sometimes more than an hour before flames appear.

Also available are interconnected "multistation" systems that trigger alarms throughout the house if smoke is detected at any ESD site.

ESDs could hardly have reached the mass consumer market at a more opportune time. Fires in houses and apartments are increasingly dangerous—about 50,000 deaths and well over a million injuries will occur because of home fires in this decade. One reason is widespread use of some synthetics and plastics that burn hotter and faster than natural materials, or that may emit toxic gases.

The National Fire Protection Association (NFPA) warns that it takes most people at least three minutes to escape the average night fire. But often the circumstances allow much less time. If you put an ESD outside your bedroom, you stand a 40-percent chance of getting that precious three-minute escape time. If you hang one on every level (including the basement), your chance rises to 88 percent.

In Scotch Plains, N.J., a family of five escaped when a teen-age son heard a new ESD wailing in a hall. The family had bought four battery-ESDs, but hung only one. As they fled, they heard bedlam in the basement: the other ESDs were sounding, *still in cartons*.

In Sacramento, Calif., five members of another family perished because they had no alarm. One shocked neighbor was pro-football player Skip Vanderbundt, husky linebacker for the San Francisco 49ers. He went out and bought a smoke detector for $70, and he and his wife Judie hung it outside their room, where it could also be heard by their two small daughters. About three months later, while Vanderbundt was on the road with the 49ers, a defective wall outlet in two-year-old Piper's room heated up and set a curtain ablaze.

The child slept on, until smoke seeping through cracks around her door triggered the ESD and brought Judie Vanderbundt bounding out of bed. Mother and girls had just reached the street when the "room flashover" that firemen dread blew up Piper's room. "Even the windows blew out," Judie says. "We'd have been dead."

How to choose your ESDs

Q. Can I start with one, then add others?

A. Yes, many do. But experts urge: If you live in a house, get that second one soon.

Q. With several dozen makes and models, how do I sort them out?

A. Two types account for most ESDs sold to date:

• Electric-eye ESDs (also called photoelectrics) "see" smoke. They have a tiny light beam which spots smoke particles coming in through holes or apertures in the detector. This type responds to any ordinary fire but is especially quick to spot those that start by smoldering. Example: TV-chair fires, which start when drowsy viewers drop cigarettes among the cushions.

• Ionization-chamber ESDs also respond to any ordinary fire, but their specialty is quick response to very small, even invisible smoke particles. Such smoke spurts from hot open-flame fires that flare up suddenly, as in wastebaskets or on curtains. A tiny trace of radioactive matter, about as much as on a watch dial, ionizes air in a small chamber, creating electric current in it. When smoke floats in, it disturbs the current and triggers an alarm.

Q. Which type is better?
A. Either can give you the critical three-minute escape time. Some experts keep *both* types in their own homes: they want the slight special advantage that each offers.

Q. How do I recognize a well-made ESD?
A. Look for the letters UL or FM. These signify successful testing by Underwriters Laboratories or Factory Mutual Research.

Q. How many do we need for a three-room apartment?
A. At minimum, one outside your bedroom door. A second unit outside your entrance could warn of *other* people's fires on floors below you.

Q. In a one-story house, can't we just get along without ESDs? It's easy to step outdoors.
A. Firemen say one-story houses seem safer but aren't. One trouble is those flashovers. Another is fire-gas that can kill you in two breaths— before you wake up.

Q. Where should the first ESD be put?
A. The No. 1 rule of fire-safety engineers is: Detect smoke before it blocks your escape routes. The preferred location is outside your

bedroom door. Additional key spots include other sleeping areas (particularly the room of any person who smokes in bed); at the top and foot of all stairs; in the front hall.

The No. 2 rule is: Protect special people in special places. So it's wise to add an ESD in the room of any child, crippled person, invalid or senior citizen.

Whether installing your ESD on the ceiling or wall, be sure to follow the instructions in the owner's manual, so that you avoid the "dead-air spaces" where ESDs should not be mounted.

Q. What about ESDs in kitchens and garages?

A. Cooking and car fumes cause too many false alarms. Even though some ESDs are advertised for kitchen use, most investigators advise a location no nearer than six feet to that room. That's close enough to detect fire quickly.

Q. I want a battery-powered unit. What do batteries cost?

A. "One-year-life" batteries cost $1.50 to $10. When they weaken, you get a signal—often it's a beep, or a warning flag that pops out.

For units permanently wired into the house current, installation costs will vary, but once the unit is installed, the electricity costs about the same as for a night light: $1 or $2 a year.

Q. Is maintenance needed?

A. Definitely yes. Vacuum ESDs twice a year to remove dust that can cause false alarms. Test each unit at least once a month (some experts say once a week). Use the built-in test mechanism, if your unit has one. Otherwise, blow the smoke of a lighted match, punk or cigarette directly into the ESD.

Q. Wouldn't false alarms be a nuisance?

A. In some homes, an electric-eye set might "false" once or twice a year, a sensitive ionization-chamber set more often. But they generally don't react when a guest lights a cigar. Some experts *like* the occasional needless alarm because it indicates that your set is sensitive enough, that it's protecting you.

One important caution: Never assume that an alarm is false and go back to bed until you've checked *thoroughly*. And even then wait awhile. One family phoned firemen that their ESD was giving a false alarm and wouldn't stop. Firemen came, found no fire, and obligingly removed the batteries from the ESD to stop the noise. An hour later the house was on fire.

PART TWO
SAFETY OUTSIDE THE HOME

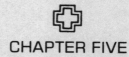

CHAPTER FIVE

HOW TO STAY SAFE OUTDOORS

What to Do
When Lightning Strikes

by G. R. von Kronenberger

WHEN A sudden storm interrupted three men playing golf in North Carolina, they retreated to a rain shelter. Moments later, lightning struck. One of the trio was completely unharmed. Another had his trousers ripped to shreds, one shoe torn off, and suffered burns on both legs. The third—though there was not a mark on his body—was dead.

By far the most destructive of nature's violent acts, lightning kills more people than any other natural disaster. Each year, it destroys property worth hundreds of millions of dollars in the United States. Few areas in this country are free of lightning storms, and the average square mile is hit by as many as 20 or 30 bolts per year. Yet much property and many lives could be saved if individuals understood this electrical force and practiced common-sense safety rules.

Lightning is an electrical phenomenon whose main charge flashes not from cloud to earth—as it sometimes appears—but from earth to cloud. When storm clouds gather, the wild turbulence inside them results in a separation of electrical charges. Usually, negative charges accumulate in the lower part of the cloud, while positive charges build up in the earth and in the upper part of the cloud. Lightning occurs when the attraction between these opposite charges becomes strong enough to bridge the gap separating them.

An imperceptible stroke "leader" advances from the cloud step by step toward the ground, establishing the path the stroke will take. When it nears the ground, an avalanche of charges rushes upward through the conducting path, reuniting positive and negative charges (or ions). This return stroke produces the brilliant flash and the clap of thunder. The leader will follow the path of least resistance. It may seek out a tree, a chimney, you—or whatever provides the shortest gap and the best conductor.

Tremendously powerful, lightning moves about 30,000 times as fast as a bullet and may contain over 100 million volts and as much as 100,000 amperes—thousands of times as much power as in your house electric current. The intense heat generated when lightning strikes directly often causes all the sap in a tree to boil instantaneously and evaporate; in a chimney, the violent expansion of the moisture in bricks may blow them into millions of pieces.

Although scientists have been unable to measure lightning precisely, its approximate dimensions are known. The core of pure electrical energy in an average bolt is about one half to three fourths of an inch thick. It is surrounded by a four-inch-thick channel of super-heated air. The length of a stroke may vary from 2000 to 15,000 feet or more and, since most lightning strokes are actually multiple, more than 40 strokes may occur in quick succession, spaced up to half a second apart.

Lightning bolts may be "hot" or "cold," or a combination of both. A hot one is a multiple stroke of long duration, perhaps as long as a second. It has high amperage and sets fire to flammable materials in its path. A cold strike is much faster, and has an explosive rather than igniting effect. A large bolt of cold lightning has enough energy to lift the 51,821-ton ocean liner *United States* six feet into the air.

The greatest number of lightning casualties, according to a study by the Lightning Protection Institute, occur outdoors, but one fourth occur in the home—mainly because that is where most people are during storms. Lightning strokes enter houses via chimneys, plumbing, wiring, TV antennas, or directly through the roof.

In one tragic case, lightning hit a tree alongside a suburban home, ran down the trunk to an attached wire clothesline, followed the line to a metal fitting that fastened it to the house, and reached a television set which touched that wall of the house. The young mother, attempting to unplug the set, was instantly killed. Her five-year-old daughter, sitting close by on a couch, was temporarily paralyzed.

A chimney with attached TV antenna—the highest point on a house—is an obvious target for lightning. The average antenna is not grounded with a large enough conductor to offer lightning protection to the house. A charge striking it may jump down the chimney or find a better conductor on the way earthward, such as metal fixtures around the fireplace or a metal heat or vent pipe. If this new conductor isn't grounded, the charge leaps out to the next-nearest conductor, and anyone happening to be in its path may get a dangerous jolt.

It is wise, therefore, to stay away from walls, fireplace, plumbing lines, electrical equipment and metal objects such as stove, sink or tub, during a storm that is striking close. Though the safest spot is generally the center of a room, see that this location does not place you between one conductor leading down from the roof and another leading to the ground. A seat between a fireplace and a metallic heating or plumbing fixture, for instance, might turn out to be an "electric chair." And since overhead telephone wires often are struck, it is a good idea to leave the telephone alone during an electrical storm.

A properly designed and installed lightning-rod system is a useful safeguard. When lightning strikes a building thus protected, the bolt is intercepted by one of the rods, then led into a heavy conducting cable which dissipates it harmlessly deep in the earth. Protection systems are neither expensive nor difficult to obtain. But be sure to employ a competent, reliable, experienced installer. This is *not* a do-it-yourself project!

The safest places to be during electrical storms are in a building with continuous steel-frame construction with the framing grounded, in a building equipped with proper lightning protection systems, or in a *closed* automobile. If you are caught in the open, do not seek shelter under isolated trees or in small groves. It is better to crouch down in the open. Best is to find a cave, ravine or ditch.

Stay away from knolls, utility poles and golf tees, and give wide berth to wire fences—their posts attract the charge, and their wires are excellent conductors. Stay out of water, and particularly out of small boats. Rocky ground in the open offers very poor conductivity for lightning current, which therefore must dissipate over a wide area. Campers should avoid such sites when pitching a tent. Also, groups of people in the open provide more attraction than individuals, and it is wise to scatter during a severe thunderstorm.

When a storm strikes so close that the flash of lightning and the report of thunder are almost simultaneous, and when the air is loaded with the pungent odor of ozone, it is time to carry precautions to the nth degree. If you are in such a storm and feel your hair beginning to stand on end, you may be getting set up as a lightning target. In such a circumstance, toss dignity to the winds and drop to a kneeling position with only your feet and knees touching the ground, and with your head down. After all, it's better to be muddy than dead.

Danger!
Stinging Insects

An interview with Dr. Robert E. Reisman

Q. Dr. Reisman, how dangerous are insect bites and stings?
A. Allergic reaction to insect stings causes an estimated 40 to 50 deaths a year in this country. And we suspect that many of the deaths from "unknown causes" that occur in summertime may also be due to insect stings. Short of mortalities, there are a large number of more common allergic reactions—generalized swelling all over the body, shortness of breath and wheezing, fainting, collapse of the vascular system, swelling of the upper airway.

Q. You say stings, not bites....
A. The stinging insects—such as bees, wasps, yellow jackets and hornets—can cause severe allergic reactions. Biting insects—ants, flies, spiders—can, but rarely do.

Q. How can a person tell if he is susceptible to allergic reactions?
A. Usually the diagnosis comes after a reaction. One might suspect susceptibility in an individual who shows progressively larger local reactions from stings.

Q. How can stings be avoided?
A. Insects are attracted by food or cooking odor, and by such things as perfumes, hair sprays, suntan lotion, cosmetics and bright colors.

We advise individuals at risk to avoid outdoor cooking or eating, and to wear light colors outside, such as whites or tans. Also, to be very careful while working outside, mowing a lawn, cutting vines, pulling weeds.

Q. What about insect repellent?
A. Repellents are not very effective in keeping stinging insects away.

Q. What should you do if a stinging insect gets in your car?
A. First, stop the car. Then roll down the windows and carefully get that insect out of the car.

Q. Are there emergency medications for individuals who have shown susceptibility?
A. Yes. And such individuals are advised to carry these medications at all times. The drug of choice is adrenalin, administered by injection; we teach individuals at risk to inject their own. Second, susceptible individuals may also be given antihistamine tablets. And because the allergic reaction occasionally may involve swelling in the throat, patients are given an inhaler which contains adrenalin.

Q. How quickly do sting reactions occur?
A. We have seen serious reactions several hours after an insect sting, but most commonly the sooner the reaction, the worse it is.

Q. For which symptoms should a victim get to a doctor at once?
A. Care should be sought immediately for almost any kind of serious reaction, including swelling of the upper airway, falling blood pressure, fainting; also wheezing, coughing and shortness of breath.

Q. How effective are immunization programs in reducing the danger of sting reaction?
A. Injections of venom solutions prepared from the actual venom of stinging insects are available and are highly effective in preventing further reactions.

Sunbathing— In a New Light

by Lowell Ponte

SUMMER HAS COME, and millions of us flock to beaches, parks and city rooftops to bathe our bodies in sunlight. For many, these doses of sunshine will bring improved health. In the right amounts, sunlight can reduce blood pressure and the levels of sugar and serum cholesterol in the blood, enhance strength, relieve asthma and aching joints, improve the uptake of oxygen in the body's cells and reduce stress.

But sunbathers who overdo it will suffer painful sunburn. Worse, their skins will lose elasticity and age prematurely. Sunburn may also damage their immune systems, impairing their defense against other injury or disease. And for more than 220,000 Americans every year, overdoses of solar radiation will eventually produce skin cancers, some of which will spread to other organs. In 1981 alone, all skin cancers claimed the lives of nearly 7000 Americans.

Why does one person tan, while another suffers sunburn? Why does a third get skin cancer? Researchers in the pioneering science of photobiology, the study of how light interacts with living things, are just now beginning to unravel the mysteries of how sunlight affects us.

More than half of the sun's radiance is invisible to human eyes. Of this, most is infrared light, so called because it vibrates more slowly than the color red at one end of the visible spectrum. We cannot see infrared radiation, but we feel it as heat.

The rest of the unseen light is ultraviolet, so named because it vibrates faster than the color violet at the other end of the spectrum. Ultraviolet is more energetic than visible or infrared light. If the earth were exposed to the full force of the sun's ultraviolet radiation, all life would quickly end. Fortunately, our planet wears a globe-encircling sunshield of gases that filter and dim incoming ultraviolet rays.

The more of this atmosphere you put between your skin and the sun, the less the ultraviolet dose. Therefore, the safest time to sunbathe is when the sun is near the horizon and its rays have to travel through more atmosphere to reach you—before 10 a.m. or after 3 p.m. in the Snowbelt, before 9 a.m. or after 4 p.m. in Sunbelt regions closer to the equator. And the safest places are low-lying areas, for the higher you are, the less atmosphere there is to shield you from the sun. For every 1000-foot rise above sea level, the dose of solar ultraviolet rays increases by five percent.

Even when dimmed by the atmosphere, the sun's rays can be dangerous to unprotected skin. Both visible and invisible solar radiation penetrate our skin's surface, smashing into living cells. This causes an electrochemical change by splitting off unpaired neutrons, called free radicals, from cell molecules. These highly reactive agents produce toxic byproducts that poison or irritate surrounding tissues and apparently contribute to the swelling and leakage of tiny blood vessels in the skin—a process we know as sunburn. They may also damage the genetic blueprints cells use in reproducing. Thus free radicals can impair cellular renewal in our bodies, hastening the aging process. Or, worse, they may cause defective cells to proliferate—a condition that can turn into cancer.

Once a cell's genetic blueprint is scrambled, it is usually unable to restore itself to health. Thus, say scientists, some of the harm done by sunlight is cumulative. With every overdose of sunlight, permanent injury is done to the body's cells.

Fortunately, our skins have an elaborate defense system against the sun's radiation. The topmost skin layer consists of flattened cells made up of a slightly yellowish substance called keratin. Beneath this layer, and its underlying special cells that manufacture keratin, lurk melanocytes, cells that produce pigment granules called melanin. The skin stores some melanin at all times. When ultraviolet rays penetrate our skin and strike the melanin, it turns dark—an automatic chemical re-action we call tanning.

A deeper tan follows as ultraviolet rays stimulate the melanocytes to produce more and more melanin. But what we boast of as a "healthy" tan is really an effort by our skin to shield itself from dangerous radiation. After several days of exposure, the dark melanin is able to absorb up to 90 percent of incoming ultraviolet radiation before the rays do further damage.

The skin has other defense mechanisms. After the first burning doses of ultraviolet rays have begun unleashing free radicals, cells in the top layers of skin begin reproducing rapidly. The skin thickens and hardens, making it more difficult for ultraviolet rays to penetrate. If even this fails and the skin flushes with sunburn, it will speed up its normal but usually unnoticed shedding—or "peeling"—of damaged and old cells.

With all these defenses, why do we get sunburned at all? The answer lies in part with our industrial civilization. If, as our ancestors did, we tilled the fields and so got some exposure to sunlight every day year-round, our skins would gradually increase their levels of protective melanin as the days lengthened during springtime. When summer came, we would be prepared. As it is, we give our winter-softened skin little chance to mobilize its defenses, to produce the layers of pigment needed for protection. Like suicidal lemmings rushing to the sea; we bare our bodies to the first warm flushes of solar radiance—and then we bear the consequences.

To compensate for this foolishness, we smear our skins with more than $200 million worth of suntan creams and lotions each year. The use of such preparations is generally wise, say doctors. But now scientists are worried that some sunscreen products may in some cases do as much harm as good.

For example, para-aminobenzoic acid (PABA) has been praised as an excellent defense against ultraviolet rays; it is used in dozens of today's most effective suntan preparations. But research in the United States and England suggests that some of PABA's chemical byproducts are phototoxins; they become poisons when struck by sunlight. Also, some people have allergic reactions to PABA; they experience burning, stinging or itching following application.

Another widely used suntan lotion ingredient used to hasten tanning,

5-methoxypsoralen, or its natural form, oil of bergamot, was last year proven by scientists to cause cancer and genetic damage in laboratory animals.

In another effort to protect themselves, many sun worshipers sport sunglasses. Yet in some cases, scientists warn, sunglasses may actually *increase* the risk of damaging the eyesight.

Doctors are finding strong evidence that exposing the eyes to ultraviolet light may result in cataracts. Just as the skin thickens and ages in bright sunlight, so, too, does the lens of the eye. As it thickens, it loses flexibility, putting a strain on the muscles that focus our vision. These stresses, plus the power of ultraviolet light itself, make the lens prone to distortion, discoloration and cloudiness.

To understand why the scientists are worried, reflect on what happens when you walk into bright sunlight without sunglasses. You squint. And the pupils of your eyes contract to protect the delicate visual receptors inside. But when you walk into sunshine while wearing improperly filtered sunglasses, your eyes *feel* protected—and your pupils remain wide-open—even though they may be in danger. For in fact many sunglasses screen out only *visible* light. Infrared and ultraviolet light are *not* being blocked to the same degree. They are burning into your eye—an eye you have unwittingly tricked into staying wide-open.

Even some foods can be a hazard in the sun. Although few sunbathers know it, certain foods—carrots, parsley and limes, for example— contain photosensitizing chemicals. When you drink a beverage containing lime juice, you increase your chances of coming in from the sun with a rash or a burn. However, foods containing vitamins A, E and C—including green leafy vegetables, whole grains and citrus fruits (except limes)—act as "free radical scavengers" and reduce the harm that the sun can do.

Drugs and other widely used chemicals may also cause photosensitivity, or even phototoxicity, in some individuals. These include many tranquilizers, barbiturates and antibiotics, birth-control pills, antihistamines, halogenated antiseptics widely used in soaps and cosmetics, and even large doses of vitamin B-2 (riboflavin).

Despite the potential harm, sunlight can be good for you—*if* you take it wisely. Sunbathe in early morning or late afternoon. Give your skin time to build up protection by sunning at first for only 20 minutes or so each day. Pay attention to the foods you eat and the medications you ingest. Above all, use common sense. Remember that the skin you save will be your own.

CHAPTER SIX

SAFETY
IN THE WATER

Secrets
To Not Drowning
in the Sea

by Peter Benchley

ON THE morning of August 21, 1973, several dozen people nearly lost their lives off Nauset Beach on Cape Cod, Massachusetts. At 11:23 a.m., lifeguard Lee Anderson had spotted a young boy in trouble and dashed into the surf, expecting that chief guard Gary Guertin would follow with a lifeline. Guertin, however, was already preoccupied with saving an elderly couple he had seen flailing helplessly in the waves. Soon the water was swarming with 50 or 60 victims—shrieking, panicked people suddenly being swept out to sea by a violent current. "The water was pouring away from the beach," Guertin later told a reporter. "It was as if someone had pulled a plug in the ocean and it was running down a drain."

Rescue teams were quickly summoned from nearby towns, and the Coast Guard dispatched an amphibious rescue craft and two helicopters. Thanks to the massive lifesaving effort, only one swimmer died, a woman whose heart gave out at Cape Cod Hospital. But an irony lingered: sudden and violent as it was, the current would have offered little threat to anyone who knew—truly knew—how to swim in the ocean.

Very few people, however, do. Though some 107 million Americans swim for pleasure, the National Safety Council believes that fewer than 12 percent of that number are competent swimmers. And good ocean

85

swimmers are a minute fraction of that 12 percent. It is a safe bet that more than 20 people a day will drown along our 12,383 miles of ocean shoreline this coming summer. Such deaths will almost always be the result of ignorance or over-confidence.

The whole key to safe ocean swimming is understanding the water. Ocean water is never still. No matter how much the ocean may resemble the classic millpond, beware: *beneath that glassy surface is a world of constant motion.*

Prevailing winds, for example, may push the waves onto the beach at an angle (waves rarely hit a beach head-on), causing a current, called a set or drift, running parallel to the beach. Unless the set is extremely fast, it shouldn't cause any worry. A swimmer should make a mental note of an object on the beach and see how quickly he is being swept away from it. The faster he is moving, the closer he should stay to shore. Never try to swim against the set; to get back to your starting point, swim *across* the set to the beach and walk back. (This theme— never swim against currents—should be stressed, for it is critical. As Gordon Howes, director of safety services for the South Pinellas, Fla., Area Chapter of the Red Cross, says, "If you like the ocean, you learn to swim with it; you never fight it.")

Most experts believe the panic at Nauset Beach was caused by a "runout." Somewhere offshore, a sandbar had built up. Millions of tons of water flowed over it toward shore. Eventually, the water level inside the bar slightly exceeded the level outside and, naturally, the water had to flow seaward. A weak spot in the bar then gave way, creating a funnel effect. Water rushed toward the opening, sweeping people with it who panicked and tried to fight it, exhausting themselves.

Runouts are quite common, and can be spotted from the beach. There will be something manifestly different about a stripe of water 15 to 50 yards wide, leading out to sea. It may be characterized by choppy, jumbled-up little waves. The water may look extraordinarily sandy or dirty or dark. Foam and bits of wood or grass will be moving seaward. (The force of runouts is negligible very close to the beach, so it poses no threat to wading children.)

A swimmer caught in a runout has a choice. He can swim parallel to the beach, across the stripe of current, until out of its power. Or he can relax and let the runout take him. He will be swept through the gap in the bar; 25 yards or so beyond it, the runout will dissipate. He can then make his way around the runout and back to shore. (Unless the bar is fairly near the beach the average swimmer should probably choose the first option.)

Another serious problem is the rip. Strong rip currents can start very near the beach and carry a child or wader into deep or rough water in seconds. Rips can be caused by a slight depression in the beach between breaking waves: the returning water will head for the depression and soon become an irresistible seaward flow. (Rips can also be caused by a set or drift being turned seaward by a pier, jetty or headland.) A rip may be very narrow at its source—anywhere from a few feet to 15 or 20 yards—and it doesn't travel as far as a runout. Usually, a rip begins to dissipate a few yards beyond the breakers. But an unsuspecting swimmer caught in one has ample opportunity to panic and drown.

The visual evidence of a rip is similar to that of a runout: a streak of turbulent, discolored water, a line of foam running directly away from the beach. The ways of coping with a rip are similar, too: swim parallel to the beach until you're free of the current, or let it take you beyond the waves until you feel its force ebb. Don't try to swim straight back to the beach. You'll never make it.

Most unknowing ocean swimmers, on arriving at an unfamiliar beach, inquire about the undertow. Also called "runback," undertow is strongest on narrow, steep beaches. Water thrown up onto the beach speeds back to sea, aided by gravity. The person who knows enough not to resist will be carried outward for a few feet toward deeper water. Then, as the next wave breaks, the undertow will cease, and he will be carried shoreward by the next incoming wave. If he *does* resist this undertow, he risks having the next wave crash down on top of him. The falling water—weighing eight pounds a gallon—may stun him, knock the wind out of him or, conceivably, in big surf, break his neck or back.

Waves are another subject many swimmers know little about. Waves don't travel in threes (or, as others believe, in fives or sevens). They travel in "trains," which can pass each other. Before you go into the water, spend a few minutes watching the waves. You may see four small waves, then one big one, then four small ones, then another big one. You're seeing one wave train overtaking another: the train of large waves has a distance between crests of, roughly, four of the smaller waves. You can know, then, that if you try to ride one of the larger waves, you'll have a time equal to four small waves in which to recover before the next big one hits you.

If you misjudge a wave and find yourself being "boiled"—that is, tumbled in a mess of froth and sand—do not obey your instinct to struggle to the surface. The turbulent water is full of air bubbles and will not support a swimmer. Relax, go limp in a curled-up, or fetal, position (a rigid arm or leg can be slammed against the bottom and snapped like a twig). Let the wave toss you around. The undertow will carry you out into calmer water where you can swim to the surface.

To avoid trouble at the beach, take a few precautions before swimming:

• Toss a small piece of driftwood into the water and see what happens to it. If it moves up or down the beach very fast, there is a strong set (drift) working.

• Wait for at least a dozen waves to break, and decide if any one of them was bigger than you'd want to try to ride.

• If you have non-swimming children, make sure that they play in the sand well above the watermark caused by the biggest wave. Wave wash is deceptively strong, and anyone playing in it should be able to swim long enough to await rescue.

• Look for rips or runouts.

• Before anybody goes into the water, make sure someone else is watching him.

• Rocky coastline and areas with fixed reefs or other obstructions may have tricky currents and wave formations. Be alert for them.

If, despite the ease with which trouble can be avoided, you do find yourself on the verge of drowning, never wave your arms over your head to attract attention—they will be heavier out of water and will cause you to sink. Instead, use the survival technique called "drownproofing," by which even marginally competent swimmers can stay afloat indefinitely. Its two premises: (1) almost everybody will float if his lungs are filled with air; (2) it is much easier and less tiring to float vertically than horizontally.

Floating vertically, with your hands limp at your sides, take a deep breath, hold it and let yourself hang there, with your face underwater. As soon as you feel that you'd like to take a breath, exhale slowly through your nose. Raise your arms and cross them in front of your face, then spread them as if you were parting curtains and, when your arms are extended, push your palms downward toward your sides and tilt your head back. Your mouth will come out of the water. Take a breath, lower your head and arms, and resume the limp, hanging posture. When you begin to feel relaxed with the technique, leisurely move your body toward the horizontal and kick toward shore.

What if you are seized by a cramp? "The important thing is not to panic," says Dr. Willard A. Krehl, president of the health maintenance program at Thomas Jefferson University Hospital in Philadelphia, who has made extensive studies of cramps. "Relax the limb as much as possible. Flex your foot toward your head, rather than extending it away from the body. Float in a way that's comfortable for you, and try to massage the muscle involved until you get relief. Some people try to use the afflicted limb, and that aggravates the cramp."

People tend to attribute malevolence to the sea, calling currents "treacherous" and waves "killers." The tendency is, I think, symptomatic of man's persistent refusal to admit that he must co-exist with nature, not try to dominate it. We should accept the sea for what it is: an environment that is different but not hostile, welcoming and rewarding to the cautious and prepared, and fatal mostly to the foolhardy.

"Rescue Breathing" The Way to Save Lives

by Richard Match

NINETEEN fifty-eight was a year of revolution in artificial-respiration methods. Experiments sponsored by the Red Cross and the Army Surgeon General showed that the best first-aid measure to revive a person whose breathing has been stopped by near-drowning, electric shock, smoke or gas inhalation, or some similarly incapacitating accident or illness is to *blow your breath into his lungs, mouth-to-mouth*. As a result, nearly every major first-aid organization in the country rewrote its official literature to make mouth-to-mouth artificial respiration— often called "rescue breathing"—the first choice in resuscitation emergencies.

The experiments demonstrated that in about half to three quarters of resuscitation cases neither the long-familiar Schaefer "prone-pressure" method nor the later recommended Holger Nielsen "back-pressure armlift" method, as usually performed by a trained rescuer, moved enough air into the lungs to sustain life. Mouth-to-mouth resuscitation, on the other hand, supplied three to four times the volume of air averaged by experts using the older methods.

No equipment is necessary for successful mouth-to-mouth breathing, and most first-aid agencies do not endorse such equipment for general use. It may not be available in emergencies, and precious seconds may be lost in searching for it.

Rescue breathing has an extra lifesaving advantage. Doctors have long recognized the danger that an insensible patient may "swallow his tongue"—and suffocate. For in an unconscious person throat reflexes

---

Be Prepared to Save a Life

Place nonbreathing victim on back, face up. To clean out any foreign matter, turn victim's head to side, force mouth open, wipe out throat and mouth with fingers or cloth.

Mouth-to-Mouth Method in Adults:

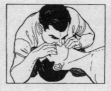

Insert thumb of your left hand between victim's teeth. Hold the jaw upward so that the head is tilted backward. Close victim's nostrils with your right hand. Take a deep breath and place your mouth tightly over victim's mouth and your own thumb. Blow forcefully enough to make victim's chest rise. Repeat inflations every five seconds.

Mouth-to-Mouth Method in Children
(or in adults with tight jaw):

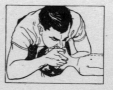

Grasp the angles of the child's jaw at the ear lobes with both hands, and lift up forcibly so that the head is tilted backward. Push child's lower lip toward the chin with your thumbs. *Never let the chin sag*. Take a breath and place your mouth tightly over child's mouth (for a small child cover both mouth and nose). Blow in gently until his chest moves, then take your mouth off and let him exhale passively. Repeat inflations once every three seconds. *For infants use puffs*.

disappear, and the tongue may sag against the back of the throat, blocking the victim's natural air passage. X-ray pictures have proven that this can happen whether the unconscious victim is placed face down or face up.

Rescue breathing avoids this danger. The victim's head *must* be tilted back and the lower jaw *must* be jutted out. The backward tilt of the head opens the victim's air passage, and the jutting jaw *pulls the tongue forward*. Authorities say that some unconscious victims will be saved simply by holding the head and jaw in this position, which permits spontaneous breathing.

Each year an estimated 14,000 Americans die of gas or smoke inhalation, drowning and similar emergencies. Three quarters of these incidents occur in or around the home. According to experts, a large percentage of the victims could be saved if everyone knew the few simple steps involved in mouth-to-mouth artificial respiration. Deprived of oxygen, brain cells die or suffer irreversible damage in as little as four to six minutes. In an emergency, therefore, start your life-giving blowing *at once*. And at the first opportunity have someone call a doctor and the most expert rescue group available.

Cold
Can Do You In

by J. Clayton Stewart

AT APPROXIMATELY 10 p.m. on December 22, 1963, fire broke out aboard the Greek luxury liner *Lakonia* as it cruised the Atlantic near Madeira, and passengers and crew were forced into the water. The air temperature was over 60 degrees, the sea almost 65, and rescue ships were in the area within a few hours. Nevertheless, 124 people died— 113 of them because of hypothermia, the lowering of the body's inner heat, perhaps by no more than six degrees.

The temperature of the hands and feet can drop 40 degrees below the normal 98.6 without lasting harm. But a relatively small drop in temperature of the body core will kill you; it makes no difference whether you're in water, the wilderness, a house out of fuel or a car out of gas. You can survive three weeks without food, and three days or so without water, but without warmth you are lucky to last three hours.

Hypothermia is a danger even in mild temperatures—say, between 30 and 50 degrees. Indeed, the majority of cases develop in this seemingly harmless range. Being wet and in the wind at such temperatures can be fatal, for the thermal conductivity of water is 32 times that of still air at the same temperature.

The moment your body begins to lose heat faster than it produces it, hypothermia threatens. According to research by the Mountain Rescue Association, the body reacts in a series of predictable ways. At 2.5 degrees below normal, shivering begins—an automatic body process to create heat. But it takes energy to shiver—comparable to what is expended sawing wood—and the heat loss continues. The more the core temperature drops, the less efficient the brain becomes. You may have a pack on your back with a sleeping bag and food in it, and not have the sense to use them.

At 95 degrees, dexterity is reduced to the point where you cannot open a jackknife or light a match. At 94, you will stop shivering, but every now and then will experience uncontrollable shaking. Your system, automatically getting rid of carbon dioxide and lactic acid, also releases blood sugar and a little adrenalin, giving you a surge of energy, which causes the violent shaking. This last desperate effort by the body to produce heat utilizes a tremendous amount of energy.

By this time, if someone were to ask you your name and telephone number, you probably wouldn't know them, for the brain has become numb. If nothing is done, death may occur as soon as 1½ hours after the shivering starts.

The speed with which hypothermia develops depends on the amount of energy available to start with. If you were warm and fresh when the plane crash-landed or the car broke down, your energy reserves may be considerable. The trick is to conserve your energy, by limiting muscular action and reducing body-heat loss.

There is no clothing that is effective in every situation. Duck down, best for stopping wind, is no use when wet. The clear plastic covering that protects against rain is not, by itself, a good insulator against cold. Wool has the peculiar virtue of drying from within, keeping the body warm even when wet. Never wear jeans when there is any possibility of exposure to cold. Loose-woven, the denim of blue jeans not only allows water to penetrate but permits wind to blow away warm air. Cotton absorbs water like a wick, and quickly becomes soaking wet.

If you find yourself without proper protection, use your wits. Lives have been saved by padding clothing with any soft, fluffy or relatively bulky material. Dry grass, moss, cattail down, and milkweed have all been used as emergency insulation. Pieces of paper packed inside your clothes are also helpful.

And protect your head. The head is the most efficient portion of the body's heating system. A person who leaves his head unprotected may lose up to half the body's total heat production. There is an old mountaineer's maxim: "When your feet are cold, put on your hat."

Dry clothing and adequate shelter are the keys to survival. But it may take too much energy to collect materials and build a shelter. It may be better to emulate the chipmunk, scooping out a body-size cave under a fallen tree where you can stay dry and insulated against the cold.

When stranded in a car or truck, stay where you are. Even after the fuel tank has run dry and the heater no longer works, you will still have a wealth of resources. An automobile has seats and insulation that can be torn up and made into sleeping bags and padding. The crankcase oil and the tires will burn. Mirrors can signal aircraft. If you resist the temptation to panic, you can remain safe and reasonably warm until help comes.

Hypothermia warning signs include intense shivering, poor coordination, stumbling, thickness of speech and loss of memory. Even mild symptoms demand immediate treatment. The ideal procedure is to wrap the victim in warm blankets and, if he is conscious, force him to drink large quantities of warm, heavily sugared liquids, or beef broth.

In the field, if symptoms of advanced hypothermia are evident, the victim should not be moved from the spot until treatment has been given. If symptoms are mild, get him into the best available shelter. Replace wet clothing with dry, and put as much insulation as you can between him and the ground. Try to keep him awake while administering liquids.

Faced with an imminent boating accident, put on warm clothing, if possible, as well as a lifejacket (experiments show that clothing can provide considerable thermal insulation, even when submerged). Once clear of the craft, float unless land is close enough to reach by swimming. Many of those who swam unnecessarily after leaving the *Lakonia* exhausted themselves, accelerating the fall in their body temperature.

In April 1967, bush pilot Robert Gauchie was discovered alive in the arctic wilderness of Canada's Northwest Territories, 58 days after he had been forced to land for lack of fuel. The 39-year-old Gauchie lost considerable weight, and his feet were frostbitten, but he was in good condition. He had existed on emergency rations and a supply of raw fish he was carrying as freight. The temperature had fallen, at times, to 60 degrees below zero, and was seldom above zero. Had he tried to walk for help, Gauchie would have perished within hours.

Few of us will ever have to face this sort of ordeal, but the rules for survival are the same. The strongest are not always the ones who live. Most likely it will be those who think clearly. Your brain is your best survival tool.

Boating Safety Is No Accident

by Jean Carper

In the summer of 1972 in Oregon, a woman joined a neighbor for a friendly run down a river in his new motorboat. Just "fooling around," he made a sharp turn; she fell overboard, and her leg was severed at the knee by the propeller.

In Ohio, several families were returning from a day of picnicking aboard a 26-foot cabin cruiser when a tow of barges loomed up ahead. The motorboat's operator apparently became confused and veered into the barges' path. The cabin cruiser was crushed and swept under the tow. Rescuers found seven bodies, including three children and the boat's operator, floating in the wreckage.

There are approximately 60 million boaters and 14 million boats in the United States today, with 400,000 additional craft put on the water each year. Given these figures, it is not surprising that accidents have become sickeningly common. Boating fatalities reached a high in 1973: 1754 dead. In 1980, the figure was 1360. During 1980 there were also more than 2600 reported boating injuries and over $16 million in property damage.

What causes boating accidents? How can they be prevented? These questions are critical to nearly everyone: to those who own and operate boats, to those who have friends and relatives with boats, to anyone who may step into a boat this summer. Here are the major types of accidents, and what can be done about them.

Capsizing and sinking.

This is the cause of about half of all small-boat fatalities. If the boat is overloaded or there are high waves, even a slight shift of weight can precipitate disaster. While trolling seven miles off the coast of Florida in a small cabin motorboat, a man hooked a fish, and his companion stepped beside him to help pull it in. Their weight lowered that side of the boat enough to allow a six-foot wave to break aboard. As the two men grabbed frantically for life jackets, the boat flipped and quickly sank. One had not had time to secure his jacket properly, and it kept coming off. His body was found the next day floating face down, with the jacket partially attached. The other man survived.

Improper loading and overloading are probably the chief factors in capsizing. The records are full of instances in which seven persons, say, set out in a boat built for three; one person moves, and the boat turns over. According to the Coast Guard, you can roughly estimate the number of people that can be safely taken aboard a small boat by multiplying its length by its width and dividing that figure by 15. (Federal law now requires that each new boat less than twenty feet—except sailboats, canoes, kayaks and inflatables—carry a capacity plate stating its maximum safe weight load.) Warns the Coast Guard: The number of seats in a boat is *not* a reliable indicator of how many people it can safely carry.

Collision.

The most frequent kind of boating injury results from one craft striking another, or a floating object, or a person. And the reason for such collisions is simple: many boat operators just don't watch where they're going. Others don't know the "rules of the road"—on which side to pass another boat, who has the right of way, how to signal intentions. (Richard Schwartz, executive director of The Boat Owners Association of the United States, suspects that many boaters do not even know there *are* such rules.)

Falling overboard.

This accounts for about 325 drownings every year. People slip while refueling or pulling up anchor, while pulling in fish or firing guns, or simply in the act of standing up. In the summer of 1972, for example, a middle-aged woman in Alabama, out fishing with her husband in a rowboat, stood up and lost her balance. As she began to fall, her husband tried to grab her, causing both of them to be dumped into the water. He tried to pull her to shore only 30 feet away, but she panicked and he couldn't keep a grip on her because of her struggling. By the time rescuers arrived, the woman had sunk out of sight.

Particularly worrisome to authorities are fishermen and hunters who fall overboard and are pulled under by heavy clothing and boots. Also implicated is alcohol: an informal Coast Guard survey estimated that 28 percent of those who fall overboard and drown are known to have been drinking.

Needless to say, most of these accidents can be prevented by heeding certain cardinal rules, the first of which is: *Never stand up in a small boat*. Also, advise authorities, don't ride the gunwales (many persons have slipped off and been swept under propellers); don't jump in to rescue someone unless all other approaches, such as throwing life preservers, extending oars, etc., have been exhausted (there are numerous cases in which the victim is saved and the would-be rescuer perishes). And remember that alcohol and boating don't mix any better than do drinking and driving a car. You can be arrested and fined for the negligent operation of a boat while under the influence of alcohol, both by Coast Guard officers and by local officials in most states.

Unsafe boats.

Although about three quarters of all boating fatalities are chalked up to "fault of operator," unsafe design or the mechanical condition of the boat may also be underlying causes. Recognizing this problem, the Coast Guard now imposes load capacity, safe powering and flotational standards for monohull boats less than twenty feet (except sailboats, etc.). Moreover, under a tough federal law, the Federal Boat Safety Act of 1971, the Coast Guard has been given authority to fine boaters from $20 to $500 for failure to carry proper equipment such as navigation lights, and to order boats off the water for "hazardous conditions" such as inadequate ventilation and fuel in the bilges.

Of course, boats do wear out and break down just like automobiles, and many accidents are attributable to such malfunctions as stalled engines, broken steering cables and fuel-line problems. A cabin cruiser exploded off the coast of Florida after makeshift repairs in the fuel system had to be made on board. In another case, a steering cable failed, causing a boat to smash into rocks.

Advises Captain Henry Lohmann, head of the Coast Guard's Boating Technical Division: "Be sure to have your boat thoroughly checked mechanically at the beginning of each boating season and at least once during the season. And be especially wary when handling gasoline. Always refuel in good light, wipe up gas spills immediately, don't smoke while refueling; after refueling, *completely* ventilate the boat for *five minutes*. Remember, one cupful of gasoline that has vaporized in a confined area has the explosive force of 15 sticks of dynamite."

No lifesaving devices.

The primary cause of drownings from boat accidents is failure to use lifesaving devices—technically known as "personal flotation devices" or PFDs. These include buoyant vests, life preservers, buoyant cushions, ring buoys. Federal law states that every boat—rowboat, sailboat, canoe, motorboat—*must* carry a U.S. Coast Guard-approved lifesaving device for every person on board. The PFDs also must be accessible—not locked away in a storage unit—and in good condition.

Even so, the law can't save you if you don't use the devices—and use them properly. All non-swimmers, children, invalids and the elderly should *wear* their jackets on board, and others should don them at the slightest sign of emergency. Make sure that they fit, are properly fastened, and provide buoyancy for the chest, not the back (which can turn a victim face down).

Although boating accidents differ in kind and cause, most are united by a common thread: ignorance. A Coast Guard survey indicated that only 20 percent of all boaters had had any kind of formal education in boat safety and handling. Novices frequently start their boats in gear, causing them to lurch forward; they anchor from the stern, instead of the bow, a maneuver which can drag the boat under; they gun their engines while approaching large waves (one cubic yard of water weighs almost a ton).

It's up to individual boaters to inform themselves, to obey the law and to take personal responsibility for their actions on water. As a Coast Guard slogan puts it: "Boating safety is no accident."

Your Spare Tire
Can Prevent a Drowning

A 23-YEAR-OLD father had just drowned in one of Missouri's state parks. A park official was explaining to the crowd that had gathered why he had been unable to save the young man. "I told him that this was a treacherous pool and that several people had drowned in it," the official said. "But he just dived right in, and since I can't swim, there was no way to save him when he got in trouble."

Most of the bystanders accepted the explanation, but a little girl spoke up. "Why didn't you go over to your car and get the spare tire to throw to the poor man?" she asked.

Adults stood speechless as the little girl went on to recount half a dozen other ways by which the park official could have saved the swimmer. The child had been taking swimming lessons, and had been taught an elementary fact which most adults have forgotten: lifesaving equipment is everywhere—if we train ourselves to recognize it.

This year some 7000 Americans will die by drowning, and perhaps three fourths of these accidents will occur in public places where rescue should be possible. There will be other people nearby who could help but fail to do so, either because they do not know what to do or because they are afraid that the swimmer, struggling to save himself, might pull them under, also.

Bystanders could be lifesavers—if they would make use of the simple things usually at hand. Consider the spare tire. Roll it into the water, and, even with the heavy steel wheel in the center, it will rise to the surface and float. The drowning swimmer—or swimmers—can hang onto it. If everyone keeps his shoulders under water, the tire will support six or seven persons.

In fact, that tire is such a good life preserver that if you swim where no lifeguard is watching, you should loosen the lug that holds the tire in place in your car, so that it will be ready for use. Then, if a swimmer gets into trouble, push the tire to him. If he is far from shore or in rough water, you can swim out to him pushing the spare ahead of you and be in no danger yourself, for you, too, can rest on the tire if necessary.

Various other objects usually present on a family outing can be used in a similar way. If you have a gallon-size Thermos jug, empty it, replace the lids, then toss the jug to a tired swimmer; or swim out with it yourself and let the swimmer hold on while he gets his breath. It will actually buoy him up a bit, and he may be able to paddle his way to safety. Or you can tow him by pulling the jug.

Any large container with a tight-fitting lid makes a good float. A foam-plastic picnic basket is extremely buoyant. Other floatable and potentially lifesaving objects found around most pools and beaches include air mattresses, foam-rubber chaise pads, beach balls, even wooden tables and benches—and, of course, life jackets, inflated toy floats and inner tubes. Even non-swimmers can push these to victims who are not far from shore.

If none of these objects is available and a swimmer is in trouble near shore or dock, you may be able to save the victim by stretching your hand out to him. But lie flat on the dock to keep from being pulled into the water yourself. You can extend your reach by using a broom, an oar, a towel, a pole, or an article of clothing. If you wade in, stand with feet apart so you won't be pulled off-balance. Even if you swim out to the drowning person, take a stick or towel or some other object so the victim will clutch it, not you.

At your own pool or beach, provide simple equipment in a convenient spot and see that all who swim there know how to use it. This will cause each of them to feel a responsibility for looking after the safety of others. The American Red Cross has developed a Farm Pond Safety Post for use in rural areas but equally recommended for lakes and home pools. This safety station is simply a thick post, not over four feet high, painted yellow and placed near the water. On the post are the words: THINK THEN ACT.

Hanging on the post are an inflated inner tube, on which is lettered FOR EMERGENCY ONLY; a 40-foot length of quarter-inch rope, securely tied at one end to the inflated tube and at the other end to a block of wood to prevent the rescuer from losing the line; and a 12- to 14-foot pole, painted white and wrapped at one end with friction tape, to extend to struggling swimmers. You might also keep a whistle for signaling in emergencies and, for lakes or ponds, a diving mask for searching for a submerged swimmer.

Remember, everyone is a life guard, and life preservers are everywhere. This summer a spare tire may save your life.

CHAPTER SEVEN

SAFETY
AWAY FROM HOME

Traveling
in Good Health

by Phyllis Wright, M.D.

"WHAT are you going to do if you get sick?" I asked two friends who were preparing last summer for an around-the-world trip.

They regarded me with surprise. "We're not planning to be sick," they assured me. "We're perfectly healthy, we're staying at the best hotels, we'll have all our shots, and we promise not to eat anything risky."

We all deplore the hypochondriac who is so preoccupied with health problems that he ruins a vacation for himself and his companions. But ignoring *all* possibility of illness can also spoil a trip. I speak with some feeling about this because I have been attacked by viruses and bacteria in the far corners of the earth. These episodes have not dimmed my enthusiasm for travel. And, because of them, my medical colleagues keep giving me the latest travel-health tips. At the drop of a passport I offer them to anyone who will listen.

A good time for that annual physical examination is a few weeks before your trip. Your doctor can then take inventory of any potential health problems and advise you how to deal with complications that might arise. If you are taking medications, be sure to take a supply to last through your trip. (If you wear eyeglasses, pack an extra pair—and carry a prescription for the lenses.)

The big question—"What shots do I need?"—depends on which

countries you plan to enter and what diseases are prevalent there at the time. In the past, to re-enter the United States everyone had to show proof of vaccination against smallpox within the past three years. This regulation no longer exists since smallpox has been eradicated. Yellow fever and cholera immunizations are still required for travel to some countries. And since jet travel has facilitated the spread of disease as well as the spread of tourists, shots for typhoid, tetanus, diphtheria, plague, polio and hepatitis—although not required—are recommended depending on your itinerary. An oral prophylactic drug is also recommended to travelers to areas with the risk of malaria. It will give you considerable peace of mind to know that if an epidemic should develop in one of the countries you have been visiting, you are both protected from the disease and spared quarantine or observation upon your return to this country.

Most immunizations should be taken well ahead of departure, so that any unpleasant reactions will not interfere with your packing and bon-voyage parties.

If you have a potentially serious medical problem, such as diabetes or severe allergies, you may wish to register with Medic Alert. Members of this non-profit organization wear a metal emblem bearing an indication of their medical problem, an identifying number and an emergency telephone number. Medic Alert maintains a 24-hour telephone service that accepts collect calls from doctors anywhere in the world, and supplies them with additional medical information. The address is Medic Alert Foundation International, Turlock, Calif. 95380.

When choosing your itinerary, preventive medical planning should play a part. Travelers with cardiac or lung problems, for example, should avoid high-altitude countries. *All* travelers should avoid trying to cover too much ground. Exhaustion is probably the biggest enemy of the tourist, so plan a day or two every week to rest up, refuel and write all those postcards you've been collecting. Observe the local customs—if the natives feel it necessary to have a siesta in the heat of the day, take one too; they know more about their climate than you do.

Some medical facts might well be borne in mind when you are selecting transportation. For example, seasoned air travelers plan extra rest periods to adjust their biological time clocks to the "jet lag" and "jet leap" problems. (T. S. Eliot said that when he flew across the Atlantic he lost three days waiting for his soul to catch up with his body.) Even the healthy traveler often finds it both mentally and physically upsetting to find that his day has become 30 hours long, or, conversely, that it is suddenly bedtime when at home he would just be sitting down to lunch. But cardiac patients may be seriously disrupted by rapid time-zone changes on jets, and may wisely choose the more gradual time changes of travel on ships or trains.

Big airlines use pressurized planes, but remember (especially if you suffer from heart trouble or lung disease) that many planes of the small feeder airlines are not pressurized at all—a fact you may become acutely aware of if you have a cold. A cold causes inflammation of the mucous membranes that may block the eustachian tubes which connect the middle ear with the throat. Thus, with rapid changes in altitude, equalization of pressure between the middle ear and the atmosphere will be delayed. The trapped air causes intense pain. Chewing gum, yawning or swallowing vigorously forces air through the eustachian tubes and may relieve the discomfort. Shrinking the mucous membranes by using inhalers or nasal decongestants may also help.

Motion sickness, which has plagued travelers since ancient times, has been largely brought under control. There are many drugs effective in combating that queasy feeling. Still, if you are apt to suffer from motion sickness, the following tips may help:

• On shipboard, arrange for a stateroom amidships near the water line, where pitch and roll are least. When on deck, fix your eyes on the horizon to minimize dizziness. Try lying down in a deck chair and putting your head back.

• Likewise, on a plane, while aloft, tilt your seat and keep your head back. Motion tests have shown that a reclining position of the head, regardless of the position of the rest of the body, is most helpful in combating motion sickness.

A common misconception is that the "change of water" is responsible for the gastro-intestinal upsets suffered by travelers. Although in some few areas water may contain enough dissolved mineral salts to exert a mild laxative effect, 99 percent of the cases of diarrhea are caused by water or food contaminated by bacteria, protozoa or viruses. Most hotels will serve bottled carbonated water on request. In addition, water may be treated with tincture of iodine or chlorine (get instructions from your local health department), or boiled. (A useful gadget is a small electric immersion heater that will boil water promptly.) Avoid putting ice in your drinks. In many countries ice blocks are dragged around on the streets or stored uncovered in alleys; they are sure to be contaminated. Also, use only safe water for brushing your teeth.

Many of us are adventurous eaters and consider new menus a large part of the pleasure of traveling. But there are rules of caution here, too. In the Orient and Mexico, avoid salads and other uncooked vegetables dug out of the ground, as in some areas night soil is still used as fertilizer. Shun rare meat since it is a sure invitation to tapeworm or other parasites. Avoid unpasteurized milk and milk products. Wherever refrigeration is a problem, stay away from custards and cream sauces, which incubate staphylococcus unless they are kept chilled.

Try not to present too many surprises too quickly to your gastrointestinal tract. If you are a meat-and-potatoes type at home, break in gradually to rich sauces and gravies and give your system a chance to adjust. And, since many fruits have a laxative effect, it is wise not to gorge on them.

Mild respiratory and intestinal problems are the most common tourist afflictions and will respond well to "tincture of time," plenty of fluids, a bland diet and rest. In the event that you become ill, call an American embassy or consulate in the vicinity for the names of physicians consulted by their staff members. In more remote areas, often Peace Corps physicians or World Health Organization medical teams can suggest a doctor.

So plan your trip carefully, take advantage of immunizations, get plenty of rest, choose your food and drink wisely, take along necessary medications—and have a marvelous time. Remember, if Marco Polo made it without any of the help you have, you ought to thrive.

Hitchhiking— Too Often the Last Ride

by Nathan M. Adams

LIKE MOST of the 200,000 other college students who live in greater Boston, Synge Gillispie, an attractive 22-year-old blonde, was a frequent—and fearless—hitchhiker. In fact, during one summer vacation she and a friend had hitchhiked across the country. On the chilly evening of November 29, 1972, however, Synge Gillispie disappeared while hitchhiking to her part-time job as a cocktail waitress in downtown Boston. Two months later, her nude and battered corpse was discovered in a wooded suburb. She was the seventh girl murdered in Boston in as many months; six of them had been abducted while thumbing rides.

• During the fall of 1972, Santa Cruz, Calif., was locked in a vise of terror. No fewer than six young women—all of them last seen hitchhiking—were victims of grisly murders. Three were decapitated; the dismembered torso of a fourth was washed ashore by the Pacific surf in January.

• At 3:35 p.m. on January 23, 1972, Lt. Joseph Pura of the Boulder, Colo., police department turned off his tape recorder and sat back in speechless horror. He had just heard the confession of Glyn Thomas Stapleton, who admitted raping more than 100 women—one every other night—in less than a year. The majority of his victims, Stapleton said, were young hitchhikers. He shot the last, 21-year-old University of Colorado co-ed Sylvia Simik, who was thumbing a ride to her part-

113

time job at a restaurant, and threw her nude body into a remote canyon.

Police and highway officials across the nation declare that violence against hitchhiking young people—particularly girls—has become a major crime wave. Indeed, statistics gathered from police in cities with high concentrations of hitchhiking students disclose a story that should be of the deepest concern to parents and students alike. For example, in Boulder in 1972, nearly 70 percent of all rape victims were hitchhikers; in Boston, 33 percent. Police in Berkeley, Calif., point out that 30 percent of the rapes committed in that city in the first two months of 1973 followed the abduction of hitchhikers.

Twenty years ago, youngsters thumbing rides were more the exception than the rule along American roadways. For the most part, the thumbers were itinerants, and it was the highway samaritan—the driver—who ran the greater risk of being robbed or assaulted.

Today, however, hitchhiking is a highly popular means of getting from here to there among young people. Often shy of funds, they point out that they cannot afford scheduled transportation. From junior high school on, students thumb lifts to and from classes as a matter of course. Others take to the highways each summer, innocent vagabonds armed with little else than a pack on their back, trust and a desire to see the country. At least a fourth of them are girls. Predictably, it is they who are the favorite prey.

In the case of a girl who hitchhikes, the odds against her reaching her destination unmolested are today literally no better than if she played Russian roulette. Police estimates, victim interviews and a polling of young hitchhikers from Boston to San Francisco reveal that one out of every six will become the victim of some category of sex crime, ranging from indecent exposure to forcible rape. Yet, in spite of this mounting evidence, girls are turning out on the roads in greater numbers than ever before. For thousands of them, the trip will end in tragedy.

Consider the case of a California girl who thumbed a ride to school with a clean-cut, well-dressed, and friendly motorist. An hour later, she was found on a deserted road, her skull and both cheekbones smashed, and a 36-inch stake driven through her chest. Incredibly, she survived. A seasoned hitchhiker, this girl was 12 years old at the time of the attack. Her assailant, a Marine now confined in a state prison, was later charged with ten other crimes against hitchhikers, and police suspect that he was responsible for many more.

Unfortunately, such violence is not uncommon. In 1972, more than a quarter of the hitchhikers victimized by sex criminals in Boston were beaten, slashed with knives or shot. One, a student nurse abducted at gunpoint, beaten and gang-raped, was so terrified by the ordeal that she was mute for two weeks.

So tempting a target is the single hitchhiker that some criminals regularly patrol roads frequented by hitchhikers—usually near cities where major universities or colleges are located. Glyn Thomas Stapleton, a prototype of today's highway rapist, was married. The father of an infant girl, he was by day a soft-spoken, hard-working telephone lineman with an unblemished record. But his was a Jekyll-and-Hyde personality. At night he would lurk near college campuses in Denver or Boulder, looking for girls thumbing a lift. It was never hard to find them.

Generally, police state that there is relatively little they can do about this new highway violence. Most hitchhike-rapists remain undetected because only one of every five girls assaulted by a motorist is likely to report it. Many young victims are embarrassed by the experience, and if not injured they prefer to avoid lengthy questioning and trial publicity.

These facts have not been lost on today's highway rapists. Already aware that the chances of being caught are slim, many weight the odds even more in their favor by preparing for their victims in advance. For example, once a young hitchhiker enters a car, she may discover—too late—that the inside door handles have been removed, effectively trapping her. Or there may be a passenger she had not seen, hiding below the level of the rear seat. After abduction, many victims are taken to locations that have been meticulously scouted and pre-selected.

But if rapists have been quick to recognize this low-risk bonanza of potential victims, young hitchhikers themselves seem to pay minimal attention to the dangers. Like a broken record, the same rationalization repeats itself over and over: "I knew that these things happened; I just didn't think they would happen to me." Their naïveté is little short of unbelievable.

In 1972, after rapes had shot up 50 percent in the area in six months,

San Diego police launched an all-out campaign to warn hitchhikers of the growing menace. Young people thumbing rides were warned by patrolmen, and were given pamphlets detailing the risks. Their names and addresses were taken, and a form letter was sent to parents requesting that they urge their son or daughter to seek a safer means of travel. Local student groups lobbied at city hall, claiming that the program restricted their freedom and mobility. The program was suspended. "What more can we do?" asks Capt. Mike Sguobba of the San Diego police.

Indeed, what more *can* be done? An outright banning of young hitchhikers from highways has frequently been suggested, and every state has some form of anti-hitchhiking legislation on its books. Police authorities believe from experience, however, that legislation is not the answer. In 1971, for example, a bill before the California legislature called for an outright ban. Petitions against it were widely circulated among students and civil-liberty groups, and enough pressure was eventually brought to bear to convince representatives that the legislation was unconstitutional. Police also point out that such a law would be more difficult to enforce than a jay-walking ordinance—and probably as ineffective. "You can imagine the problems," says one patrolman. "I'd be arresting kids right and left. There'd be so many of them you'd have to set up a separate traffic court."

Since laws don't appear to be the answer, one alternative would be to improve transportation facilities on city campuses—a favorite haunt of hitchhike-rapists—so that students would not need to commute to class by thumb. Unfortunately, many college officials are reluctant to move in this direction. But, after a San Diego State College co-ed was raped and murdered by a motorist, one faculty member decided to take matters into his own hands.

Jack Haberstroh, an associate professor in the college of professional studies, discovered that most hitchhike-rapes occurred along a stretch of highway heavily traveled by students commuting between the college and off-campus housing. He then went out and purchased two ancient buses, which he remodeled to look like caterpillars and supplied with taped rock music and free snacks. Nicknamed the Bug Line, Haberstroh's bus service was an instant hit with students, and shuttled nearly

100 students every day. Many of them would otherwise have been hitchhiking.

Although colleges whose campuses are plagued with sex criminals would be wise to follow Haberstroh's example, an upgrading of bus services near universities can be only a partial solution to this wave of violence. Two other steps that could be taken immediately would be helpful.

1. Overwhelming evidence indicates that most victims do not report the crime because of the embarrassment of red-tape investigation and trial. Trials should be speedy and closed to voyeur-spectators. Judges should also limit tactics employed by some defense attorneys, whose cross-examinations of victims are probing, brutal, and frequently irrelevant.

2. Brochures, packed with the chilling statistics of hitchhiking hazards, should be made available to students from junior high school through college, to their parents, and to school administrators.

TRAGICALLY, many young people, confident of their own invulnerability, will continue to hitchhike no matter how appalling the risks. Before they extend their thumbs for the next free lift, however, let them pause to consider the Synge Gillispies, the Sylvia Simiks, and those last, terrible moments when these girls knew they were going to die. For them, and for too many others like them, that free ride was the most expensive ride of all.

Is Your Child's School Safe From Fire?

by Don Wharton

ON DEC. 1, 1958, 92 children and three teachers lost their lives in the tragic fire at Our Lady of the Angels School in Chicago. Many died at their desks, others in desperate struggles at blocked exits. And 76 more boys and girls were seriously injured, many crippled or scarred for life.

Two years later, almost to the day, fire broke out in St. Joseph's School in Kingston, N.Y., a building of almost identical construction. The flames started in a paper-filled basement storage room connected by an open doorway with the school's boiler room. Overhead were wood floors supported by dried-out wood joists, all sitting at the base of an open wooden stairway. It was a setting for horror. Yet when the first fire truck rolled up, 421 pupils and their teachers were completing an orderly evacuation. There were no injuries, and the fire was out, completely extinguished by water from two sprinkler heads.

These sprinkler heads in the storage-room ceiling had done three things: The first one, activated by the heat, had opened a valve that caused bells to ring throughout the school, starting the evacuation. Simultaneously, it had set off an alarm at fire-department headquarters. Meanwhile, the sprinkler head, along with a now-activated second head, was pouring 40 gallons of water a minute on the flames, controlling not only the fire but, more important, the dangerous fumes and smoke before they could spread up the stairs.

118

St. Joseph's was one of hundreds of schools that took a second look at safety measures after the fire at Our Lady of the Angels, and installed automatic sprinkler systems. At thousands of others, however, complacency and penny-pinching gradually set in after the initial shock, and nothing substantial was done to improve fire safety. From 1960 through 1968, the annual number of school fires increased from 3000 to 7900.

In 1963 a fire in a Long Island school blocked a stairway with smoke and trapped hundreds of pupils on the second floor. They headed for a window at the end of a corridor, but found it equipped with fasteners that kept the sash from being raised more than nine inches. The window was smashed, and blood streamed down the building as terror-stricken teen-agers gashed themselves squeezing through. Fourteen who didn't get out were rescued, unconscious, by firemen. This fire originated in an attic above the auditorium—there were no sprinklers to knock it out.

Only about five in 100 schools have complete sprinkler systems, and when new schools are planned, sprinklers are often quick to be eliminated because it is thought that total building costs will be higher than estimated. Almost as bad are the schools that have tried to save money by installing partial sprinkler systems covering only "hot spot" areas, such as boiler rooms, storage rooms, labs and workshops. This is hedging with children's lives.

"Don't try to guess where fires will start," the National Fire Protection Association urges. Over 35 percent of our school fires start in classrooms and school offices—the very places usually left uncovered by partial sprinkler systems. Even in the most modern building you cannot have complete safety without sprinklers. In 1967, a six-million-dollar Wisconsin high school, considered fireproof by school officials, had a night fire that destroyed six classrooms, a storage room and the school's 9000-volume library; the flames fed on furnishings, supplies and ceiling materials. In one "fire-resistive" school I found the furnace room crammed with large ash cans full of trash. The trash alone, said the fireman accompanying me, could generate enough smoke and gas "to kill every child in this school."

It takes amazingly little fire and smoke to kill. Fire inspectors have proved that if the combustibles in an average classroom were placed in an absolutely fireproof multi-story school building and ignited, sufficient heat, smoke and gas would be produced to kill most, if not all, of the classroom's occupants. What's often overlooked is that while the children in that room might escape, the fire, if not controlled by sprinklers, could produce fumes fatal to children in other classrooms.

Over 75 percent of school fires occur when no one is in the building, and most are the result of arson. Many schools are installing detection systems these days that transmit an alarm to the fire department. But why not a sprinkler system that does that and pours water on the fire, too? In New Orleans, in August 1968, when school was not in session, a fire was started by a child lighting papers in the corner of a classroom. The sprinklers responded, and damages totaled $316. Four months later, during Christmas holidays, an incendiary got into a similar New Orleans school that had no sprinklers; damages totaled $75,000. While professional arsonists know how to immobilize a sprinkler system, if a schoolboy attempts anything like that he'll actually cause the system to alert the fire station.

Each year school-fire losses are over $100 million—enough money to put complete sprinkler systems in *billions* of dollars worth of new school buildings. And consider insurance savings, particularly in areas with volunteer fire departments.

In the fall of 1968, a $3,200,000 junior high school was built in a consolidated school district of New York State and fully equipped with automatic sprinklers at a cost of $29,785. The school's fire-insurance rate was two cents per $100, compared to the 13 cents it would otherwise have been. The yearly savings of $3520 have now more than paid for the sprinkler system (including all interest).

Adding to the logic of sprinklers is the fact that schools are as liable as individuals to negligence suits. Financial losses from such suits can dwarf the property losses. For instance, in the Our Lady of the Angels fire, the building was worth only about $100,000; the total payments to parents of the dead and injured came to $3,200,000.

Some school superintendents defend lack of sprinklers by noting that they are "complying" with state or local fire codes. But many codes are outdated and should be revised.

I live in New York City, which has done a great deal to improve school-fire safety, including installation of partial sprinkler systems in all public schools. Yet it still has no "completely" sprinklered public school among its 1100 structures, and finds it necessary to operate some 30 ancient "non-fireproof" buildings.

Sizable steps have been taken by other cities to get extra protection. Chicago has put complete sprinkler systems in 230 schools. Los Angeles has spent $7.5 million putting broader-than-usual partial sprinkler systems in its older buildings. Its policy is two-pronged: to build new schools without any interior corridors or interior stairways, generally of one-story construction, with every classroom given two exits directly to the outdoors; to protect existing buildings with sprinklers that cover not only the obvious "hot areas" but also all corridors, stairways, laboratories, art rooms, etc.

It would be too much to say that sprinklers should be installed in every school, without exception, including the new Los Angeles types. But a school without sprinklers should make you think.

If your child's school doesn't have them, the burden lies upon the school authorities to explain why not. If they can't do this, your child may be in grave danger.

CHAPTER EIGHT

SOME
ENVIRONMENTAL HAZARDS

Watch Out
For Electric Smog

by Lowell Ponte

ON A MOONLESS NIGHT in upstate New York, townspeople carrying eerily glowing glass tubes rally beneath a new ultrahigh-voltage power line. "We're scared," says one. "There's enough electricity in the air 200 feet from those wires to light these fluorescent bulbs. We want scientists to find out if living near this kind of radiation causes cancer."

• In Massachusetts, Cape Cod residents file a lawsuit to halt completion of a giant U.S. Air Force radar station until studies can prove that its microwave radiation will not harm people nearby.

• In Michigan's Upper Peninsula, voters overwhelmingly reject a U.S. Navy plan to build a high-power radio transmitter. They fear the unknown effects this transmitter's intense signal might have on wildlife and people.

At issue is electromagnetic pollution—"electric smog"—the unseen energy waves that spread outward like ripples in a pond around every electrical device we use. And we use many. The United States is wired with half a million miles of high-voltage power lines. For communications we depend on 250,000 microwave relay links. Airliners see and are seen via radar. Nine million broadcasting transmitters and microwave relay stations, and 30 million CB radios flood our airwaves. Industry employs 35 million electromagnetic devices. Americans relax in the electron phosphorescence of 125 million TV sets. Eight million families cook with microwave ovens. As a result, a typical American now gets a daily dose of electromagnetic radiation up to 200 million times more intense than what his ancestors took in from the sun, stars and other natural sources.

"It feels like a spider crawling on you," says Marilyn Gruber, describing the sensation of being underneath a 765,000-volt (765 kilovolt) line that utility companies began operating across her Minnesota farm in 1978. "You can hear it, you can feel it," says her husband Werner, "but you can't see it."

Standing 50 feet below such wires, you become "coupled" with a 10,000-volt-per-meter electromagnetic force field. You can hear the crackle of air being cooked into ozone, a molecule found in smog. Energy within the field can burn leaf tips of plants under the line. It can send a painful spark jumping between your hand and a nearby tractor. Hairs on your scalp and arms twitch from the electrical forces at work.

The energy waves emitted by most power lines, along with radio waves and microwaves, have long been thought harmless (except in doses intense enough to heat tissue, as in a microwave oven). New research indicates, however, that exposure to levels of electric radiation once called safe produces disquieting results. Consider:

Andrew Marino, a biophysicist at the Veterans Administration Medical Center in Syracuse, N.Y., has studied people and animals exposed in laboratory experiments to electric smog simulating that around high-voltage power lines. "Exposure levels like those under the wire can cause a stunting of growth," Marino reports. "Levels like those 300 to 500 feet away cause physiological effects such as changes in blood chemistry and heart rate. At 1000 feet there are behavioral effects such as drops in human reaction time."

In 1973, W. Ross Adey, in experiments at the Brain Research Institute at UCLA, exposed laboratory monkeys to electric radiation of frequencies that are present around us every day. The monkeys' behavior changed and their sense of time was distorted.

Adey believes that electric smog alters our natural biological rhythms, the internal clocks that regulate waking and sleeping and thousands of more subtle body processes. The earth's magnetic field and other naturally occurring, rhythmically varying fields influence the way all living things synchronize their internal clocks. Power lines create artificial electromagnetic force fields that override this natural magnetism. According to Adey, we respond by adjusting our biological rhythms to the pulse of electric smog. This may put stress on the body. Result: general resistance breaks down, and a person may fall victim to diseases he otherwise would have fought off. This may explain why, according to University of Colorado medical researchers, the death rate for certain cancers such as leukemia is higher than average in homes within 130 feet of high-current power lines.

Still, on the whole, Americans have done little research on electric smog. The Soviets, however, have done much. Hundreds of Russian and Eastern European experiments have shown that electromagnetic fields may cause a host of health problems, including hypertension, heart attacks, headaches, sexual dysfunction, drowsiness, nervous exhaustion and blood disorders.

As a result, the Soviet Union has strict rules over the amount and duration of microwave emissions from radio transmitters and radars a person can safely absorb. The United States, by comparison, has no legal restriction for electromagnetic-radiation exposure, only an informal guideline. Set in 1966 by the U.S. American Standard Institute, the guideline calls safe any dose not exceeding .01 of a watt per square centimeter of exposed flesh (one-tenth the intensity at which microwaves are assumed to create heat). The Soviet criterion is 1000 times tougher than this for workers, 10,000 times tougher for civilians. Clearly, the Russians believe even small doses of electric smog, over time, can do great harm.

But did they believe it in 1962? That year, the CIA discovered that the Soviets were beaming radar-like microwaves into the U.S. embassy in Moscow. The radiation was .002 of the intensity the American guideline calls dangerous, but it was deliberate, aimed at the office of the U.S. ambassador from two buildings across the street.

The CIA set up experiments to duplicate what is named the "Moscow Signal." Monkeys were irradiated at the same frequencies and intensity as the embassy. Within three weeks there were adverse effects on the animals' nervous and immune systems.

Embassy personnel were not informed of the irradiation. Instead, they were asked to give blood samples to "test for a disease in Moscow's water." The tests revealed that a third had white-blood-cell counts almost 50 percent higher than normal—often a symptom of severe infection and also a characteristic of leukemia.

In 1976, the U.S. State Department declared the Moscow embassy an "unhealthful post," and metal window screens were put up to shield against the microwave beams. But 14 years had already gone by. Today, those former embassy personnel exhibit a higher rate of cancer than the American average, and two U.S. ambassadors in Moscow subjected to this microwave radiation have died of cancer. Whatever its purpose, the Moscow Signal stopped suddenly in May 1979.

In 1968, the U.S. Navy announced plans to build an extraordinary radio system in northern Wisconsin. Called Project Sanguine, it was designed to assure that the President can communicate with our undersea submarines in the event of war. A massive antenna would be buried under 25,600 square miles of countryside, and into this antenna giant transmitters would pump 30 million watts of power. The resulting signal would vibrate through the earth at a level close to the 60-hertz alternating current of American power lines and household wiring.

Environmentalist protests prompted the Navy to move its plans for Project Sanguine to Texas in 1973, where more objections blocked construction.

Meanwhile, in northern Wisconsin the Navy began operating a miniature version of Sanguine to prove the project's efficacy and safety. Studies of the system seemed to show mixed results, but in 1977 the American Academy of Science validated the safety and environmental compatibility of a modified Extremely Low Frequency System (ELF). In late 1981, President Reagan approved the recommendation to proceed with an ELF communication system having transmitters in Michigan and Wisconsin. The Navy and independent researchers say that there should be no hazard from the ELF system, and they plan to continue to monitor its use, but if there are long-term effects from exposure, we may not know until it is too late.

WHAT, THEN, can people do to protect themselves against the dangers of electric smog?

1. We must sort out the jumble of more than a dozen government

agencies, each of which claims some authority over electromagnetic radiation. In 1979, Rep. Elizabeth Holtzman (D., N.Y.) asked the White House to take responsibility for government policy and oversight.

2. The government must increase funding of independent, objective research that includes participation by scientists concerned with electromagnetic radiation. In the past, studies by utility companies, the military and environmentalists have been ignored or attacked because their results were labeled biased.

3. On the basis of research findings, we must urge the government to establish *legal* safe standards for exposure to and emission of electric radiation.

4. We must encourage putting high-voltage lines underground, however costly the process may be. Thus shielded, their electromagnetic smog will pose less of a hazard. Tax incentives could be offered to companies that bury their cables.

5. We must limit electric smog through state and local action. For example, often television and radio transmitters sit atop tall buildings in city centers, and federal Environmental Protection Agency measurements show that they heavily irradiate people in nearby tall buildings and on the streets below. When EPA tests declared Portland, Ore., one of the electrically "smoggiest" cities in America in 1976, citizens blocked construction of a new television transmitter. Oregon's legislature is considering a law to make electromagnetic polluting a crime.

STEPS such as these will help to reduce hazards posed by electric smog. Just as cave dwellers discovered and only later learned to live safely with fire, we must learn to handle radiant electricity with greater care.

Warning: X Rays May Be Dangerous to Your Health

by Fred Warshofsky

EACH YEAR, more than 130 million Americans are exposed to over 200 million medical and dental X-ray examinations, involving the taking of some 700 million films. Such X rays make up 90 percent of all the man-made radiation to which we are exposed, and undoubtedly save hundreds of thousands of lives each year. At the same time, however, experts have become increasingly concerned that X rays may pose a threat to the genetic inheritance of children as yet unconceived and that they may be causing a significant number of avoidable cancer deaths each year. Shockingly, many diagnostic X-ray exams, about 30 percent, according to John Villforth, director of the U.S. Food and Drug Administration Bureau of Radiological Health, are unproductive—the examinations must be repeated because of poor technique or weren't medically needed in the first place.

Medical X rays are packed with tremendous energy. The beams rip like lightning bolts through the delicate walls of cells, altering their metabolism, changing their character, often destroying them. If enough cells of a particular type are damaged, the results can be disastrous. If, for example, they are blood-making cells in the bone marrow and enough of them are damaged, leukemia could result. K. Z. Morgan, former director of the Health Physics Division, Oak Ridge National Laboratories, estimates that deaths due to diagnostic X-ray-induced diseases (such as bone cancer, thyroid tumors and leukemia) range from 4000 to 130,000 annually, with his most probable lowest estimate at 15,000.

The threat to our reproductive cells is also causing concern. If these cells, housed in the male and female genitals, are damaged by X rays, the chances of genetic defects in the offspring—from slightly increased susceptibility to certain chronic diseases, such as high blood pressure, to a host of lethal mutations—are greatly increased.

No one knows precisely how much of a radiation dose will cause mutations. But animal experiments have convinced radiation biologists that *any* dose to the gonads—no matter how small—carries some risk. The effects, furthermore, are cumulative. K. Z. Morgan estimates that as many as 30,000 malignancies, stillbirths and spontaneous abortions may occur each year in future generations because of such genetic damage. One study indicates, for example, that there may be increased risk of childhood cancers as a result of X-ray exposure of the mother prior to conception. This means that the reproductive machinery of the mother had been altered by X rays in such a way as to include an increased risk of cancer as part of the future child's genetic inheritance, and henceforth this inheritance may be passed from one generation to another.

Perhaps the greatest X-ray threat comes during pregnancy. A Harvard study of more than 700,000 infants in 39 U.S. hospitals showed a 40 percent increase in leukemia and cancer of the central nervous system in children whose mothers' abdominal areas were X-rayed during pregnancy. A study in Great Britain by Dr. Alice Stewart found that the risk of leukemia and other forms of cancer is about 50 percent higher among children whose mothers received abdominal X rays during pregnancy. As a result of such findings the International Commission on Radiological Protection recommends that all radiological examinations of the lower abdomen and pelvis of women of reproductive capacity, that are not in connection with an immediate illness of the patient, be limited to the ten-day interval following the onset of menstruation, the period when pregnancy is least likely. Yet pregnant women are still being exposed to X rays in the pelvic area.

Why are people subjected so needlessly to X rays? One trouble is that too many X-ray machines in the United States are owned and operated by non-radiologists (such as general practitioners, dentists and chiropractors), who have little education in health physics or radiation protection. Only 14 states require that X-ray technicians be licensed, and 13 of those exempt the physician simply because he has an M.D. after his name. But many medical-school curricula have no more than two or three lectures on radiological protection and techniques. Actually, the only real X-ray training the non-radiologist gets is more than likely from the X-ray-equipment salesman, who may well be more interested in selling machines than in protecting the patient.

But in many instances radiation protection is easy to provide. For example, according to FDA regulation, X-ray machines made after 1974 must have a device called an automatic collimator, which narrows the X-ray-beam size to the exact size of the film. Without collimation, the beam is often as much as four times larger than necessary, thereby exposing far more of the body area. In the case of chest, abdominal and spinal X rays, this means that the gonads are also irradiated. What about machines made before 1974? Although they do not have automatic collimators, they do have manually adjustable ones that can do the same job, if the operator is careful. "Manual collimation means that the beam must be aimed more precisely," explains John Villforth. "If the doctor or technician is careless about aiming and adjusting the collimator, he may miss the target organ entirely and have to reshoot. Too many are willing to expose the patient to a lot more beam, to be certain of getting their picture."

Another way to reduce or eliminate X-ray exposure of the gonads is to use special lead shields over the reproductive organs during X rays of the abdomen or lower back. This is easy to do for male patients, but sometimes impossible for females. The location of the ovaries in the abdomen means that the shield sometimes would obscure needed parts of the X-ray picture.

The best way to reduce exposure, obviously, would be to eliminate unnecessary X-ray examinations. Why are they made? Sometimes the patient pressures the doctor into ordering an X ray because he feels that an examination is incomplete without one. Sometimes physicians are so fearful of malpractice suits that they will order X rays simply to have evidence to show the nature of the problem treated and that their treatment was correct. Sometimes, with Medicaid and local programs paying $7 to $40 for a common X-ray procedure, doctors and dentists use their machines simply to make money. It is suspected that in some ghetto clinics, even before seeing a doctor, patients have two chest X rays, a spinal X ray for the chiropractor and two X rays of the feet for the podiatrist. Later the patient may have a full set of 14 mouth X rays made for the dentist. In New York one dentist with 17 X-ray machines in his two offices sued Medicaid for non-payment of more than $300,000 in X-ray fees.

But it is in the daily practice of medicine that most people are needlessly exposed, simply because X rays have become routine. "It is," said Dr. John L. McClenahan in an editorial in *Radiology*, "easier to order an X-ray examination than to think." Proving this point, Drs. Russell S. Bell and John W. Loop of the University of Washington School of Medicine studied 435 patients who received head injuries and were X-rayed in hospital emergency rooms even though preliminary examination did not indicate a fracture. They did not find a single patient whose treatment was significantly different as a result of X ray. Bell and Loop found that 34 percent of the skull X rays were made for legal reasons, anticipating a suit or insurance claim.

Considerable progress is being made in reducing the routine use of X ray. Such old routines as mass chest X rays are being eliminated. But too many dentists still routinely X-ray their patients whether or not a clinical need exists. With the help of the Bureau of Radiological Health, physicians are gradually establishing guidelines as to when certain X-ray exams are needed and when they're not. The single most important step, however—the enforcement of standards for everyone who operates X-ray equipment—is the province of the states, and the majority of states have not yet established any standards.

For all its dangers, the X ray is certainly too important a tool to abandon. Until everyone who operates X-ray equipment is properly trained and made to conform to standards, there are questions the patient himself can ask to prevent unnecessary exposure. He should ask his physician or dentist:

• "Is this X ray really needed?"
• "Are there no previously made X-ray films or other test results that

might provide the needed information?" (It's a good idea for the patient to keep a record of all his X rays.)

• "If the X ray is essential, has every step been taken to limit the exposure to the absolute minimum, to restrict the X-ray beam to that part of my body undergoing examination, and to shield my reproductive organs if that's appropriate?"

If everyone who operates X-ray equipment will proceed only when he can answer yes to these questions, then the X-ray beam will continue its role as a vital weapon against disease and not itself become a threat to health.

PART THREE
STAYING ALIVE ON THE ROAD

CHAPTER NINE

PRINCIPLES OF SAFE DRIVING

How To Stay Alive on the Highways

by James Nathan Miller

IN THE 1960s, Americans roaring along turnpikes at 65 m.p.h. were thrust into a new kind of driving environment: what the Institute of Traffic Engineers calls "the freeway situation." But too few of us are aware of the importance of adapting our driving procedures to the requirements of these highways. As a result, some of our ingrained habits, less hazardous on the old roads, are today killing and injuring thousands on the expressways.

Probably the safest drivers are the people who are in a position to learn from our mistakes: traffic engineers, safety researchers, highway patrolmen and police-science instructors. The techniques these experts use for staying alive on the highways result from what they have absorbed from analyzing grisly killed-and-maimed statistics, or re-engineering a road to prevent cars from careering off it, or sweeping the blood and shattered glass off the same stretch of highway month after month. Here are some of the most important lessons.

Many fatal freeway accidents are caused by two old familiar nuisances: getting a flat or running out of gas. Modern roads are designed almost like air lanes—to keep traffic moving fast, smoothly and *without stops*. You're safest when moving along at the speed of the general flow. When you do stop, with a steady stream of one- to two-ton metal missiles hurtling past you, you're in mortal danger if there is no shoulder to drive onto.

Consider a case that happened on the New Jersey Turnpike: A car had a flat tire on the Passaic River Bridge. There was no shoulder, so the driver had to stop in the travel lane. As his passenger walked ahead for help, the driver impatiently began changing the left rear tire by himself. He was killed by a truck.

Thus the first rule of expressway driving is to check your gas and tires before you set off on a trip. If you must stop on an expressway, get as far off onto the shoulder as possible and wait for help. If there is no shoulder, *immediately* turn on your four-way emergency flasher and get all passengers out of the car on the side away from traffic. Go back along the side of the road waving traffic off. Don't stop until you're several hundred feet behind your auto, and keep waving cars away until the police arrive. Furthermore, if you see somebody stranded like this, don't stop; notify the first readily available policeman or toll collector.

One habit that is lethal on expressways is the failure to map a route in advance. In the tourist season, when the number of out-of-state drivers increases, accidents skyrocket at the interchanges of interstate highways. What happens is this:

A man in New York City sets off for a town—say, Windsor Locks, Conn., halfway between Boston and New York. For the first few miles, interchange signs read, "New England," and he knows that he is headed in the right direction. But suddenly, as he gets closer to his destination, he's confronted—in heavy traffic—with a sign reading, "Boston Right, Springfield Left." But which way to Windsor Locks? He must make the correct decision instantly.

Those few seconds of decision are chaos: hesitation, changing lanes, a last-minute swerve or, most dangerous of all, stopping and *backing against traffic* to reach the exit. Traffic engineers agree that chances of surviving this maneuver are no better than 50-50.

Over half of all expressway accidents are at the highway "points of decision." Countless studies have been made by traffic authorities on how best to "sign" a road at these points, to satisfy the needs of local drivers, through travelers and strangers looking for exits. Many expressway exits are designed to run parallel to the main road for long distances, so that the motorist has ample warning of the exit and can slow down in the deceleration lane, instead of on the main highway.

But the best solution is for the driver to prepare himself for decision points by studying a road map before starting his trip. Even then, if you find that you must make a last-minute decision to turn off a turnpike, *don't*. Keep going with the traffic stream, even if it adds 50 miles to your trip.

Another hazard of the freeway situation is the rapid increase of high-speed, chain-reaction pileups—sometimes involving 20 or 30 cars. To help drivers avoid this, the don't-tailgate rule needs an added sentence: Don't *be* tailgated. Highway patrolmen constantly see chain-reaction accidents in which one driver, following at a safe distance, breaks the chain—only to have another chain started by a tailgater who slams into *him*.

To prevent this, one state trooper has adopted what he calls his "sandwich theory" of high-speed driving. He concerns himself with the total distance between *three* cars, with his the center of the sandwich. The closer the driver behind him tailgates, the farther he drops back of the driver ahead, to give both himself and the tailgating car sufficient room to glide to a crashless stop.

Probably the most striking difference between the old and new roads is psychological. Studies conducted by the Bureau of Public Roads in 1962 show that drivers are about three times as tense on a city street as on a freeway. As a result, they let their guard down on a thruway. James Slavin, former director of Northwestern University's Traffic Institute, has said "You see it all the time—a driver bowling along an expressway with one arm draped over the back of the seat, while three fingers of the left hand do the steering." The quietness of the motor in today's cars conspires with the smoothness of the new roads to multiply the danger. It's all too easy to drift up to 70 without any change in engine noise to warn you of the higher speed.

Maj. Robert Quick, former head of the New York Thruway's state-police patrol, gave this advice for thruway driving: "When the road looks so safe that you think you can relax, don't." The reason is obvious: at expressway speeds the reaction-time margin of safety shrinks from seconds to fractions of a second. The slightest deviation from normal conditions—a hot cigarette ash falling on a driver's hand, a squirrel darting in front of traffic—can turn a smooth-flowing stream into a pile of jagged steel and severed limbs.

Experts have a sixth-sense alertness to trouble ahead. They know that accidents tend to occur at certain kinds of universal danger spots, and they've learned to recognize the advance warnings of such high-accident-frequency locations.

When an expressway sign indicates an upcoming interchange, for instance, they switch to the lane opposite to where the two streams of traffic will be meshing or unmeshing. Then they allow extra distance between their car and the one ahead in case the other driver suddenly decides to turn off. Finally, they keep especially alert to car movements ahead and to the right (where most new expressway exits are), for they know that sudden "marginal friction" on one side of the road can almost instantly spread havoc to the other side as cars swerve away from a danger spot.

One of the most valuable techniques for safe driving is to be able to spot signs that have been installed *as a result of accidents on a given stretch*. The sign, "Deer Crossing," for instance, is usually ignored by ordinary drivers.

In 1981, ten percent of the New York Thruway's 4724 accidents were caused by deer. Traffic engineer Arthur Freed, who was himself badly injured when his car collided with a deer, advises: "When you see a deer sign, always scan the borders of the road. Deer travel in families. The deer that I hit came across the road after I had already seen three go by. At night in deer territory, use your bright lights to provide a wider off-the-road view."

The sign which many experts respect the most is "Slippery When Wet." Even on a road dampened only by a light sprinkle, they assume that if they applied the brakes suddenly, their car would react as it would on glare ice. Indeed, a few raindrops can make a road skiddier than a downpour because of oil buildup; a sprinkle causes the oil to form slippery little beads, while a heavy rain washes away oil film. The road condition most dreaded by highway authorities is a long drought (during which the oil slick builds up) followed by a light sprinkle. One summer such a combination produced one of New York's worst rashes of skidding accidents.

Basically, the lesson our mistakes have taught the experts is this: if you know what *can* happen, and then drive as if it *will*, the chances are much greater that it *won't*. This is how they stay alive.

Tailgating—
Invitation to Tragedy

by Paul W. Kearney

"IF HE HAD chased me with a shotgun or butcher knife, they'd have called it manslaughter and had him up before a jury. But he just chased me down with a two-ton car, killed my wife and son and put me in the hospital, and they called it an accident and let him go."

This, spoken from a traction bed in New England, was one victim's bitter indictment of the kind of driving known as "tailgating"—the practice of driving too close to the car ahead, even though experience and common sense indicate that any emergency stop would require a far greater margin of safety.

This indictment is your concern. Within a year over 2000 Americans will be killed in accidents involving rear-end collisions, many of which are caused by tailgating.

In 1965, Federal Highway Commissioner Rex M. Whitton estimated that rear-end collisions (including same-direction sideswipes) accounted for 46 percent of all daytime accidents in the United States. Both Pennsylvania Turnpike and New Jersey Turnpike officials reported that the rear-end collision had been far and away their leading accident. The National Safety Council said that tailgating is reported in 13 percent of all smashups.

The resulting cost and carnage are truly prodigious. Shortly before Christmas in 1962, a woman driver pulled partway off the Santa Ana

Freeway in California with a flat tire. A driver slowed to get around her and a following car smacked him. This set off a chain reaction that piled up cars for two miles. One person was killed, 24 were hospitalized, and 25 others were injured. Of the 200 cars involved, 20 were demolished and 40 disabled. "We were bouncing off each other like pingpong balls," said one driver.

We don't need to put up with this sort of accident. It is not a price we have to pay for driving. We can cut the toll—by half, by three quarters. How? I have some suggestions.

Think bigger.

I recently asked several drivers how closely they could safely follow another car at 65 miles an hour. "Two hundred feet," said one. "Two car lengths," said another. It's a wonder they're still around. The old rule of thumb is that you should stay one car length behind the car ahead for each ten miles an hour of speed. The National Safety Council now recommends the two-second rule. When the driver ahead of you passes a marker, such as a light pole or a shadow on the road, begin counting, from the back of his vehicle to the front of yours: one thousand one, one thousand two. You should not reach the mark before you finish counting. If you do, slow down and try again.

Why do you need all this distance between you and the car ahead? Because, despite what you may have heard, today's cars won't stop on a dime. Moreover, there are delays called perception time and reaction time. It normally takes you ¾ of a second to 2 seconds to perceive that there is trouble coming when the car ahead suddenly begins to slow down. And it takes you more time—another ⅕ of a second—to get your foot off the accelerator and onto the brake. Thus at 55 you travel at least 76 feet before your brakes even begin to take hold.

Keep moving.

A young woman recently rolled up an approach to the Merritt Parkway in Connecticut, saw a break in the onrushing stampede of traffic and moved in. But she was a cautious type, not given to quick acceleration or speed, and even after 200 yards on the 55-mile-an-hour parkway she was moving at only 45. Cars piled up behind her, tires screeched, someone tried to change lanes, and when it was over three persons were injured and two were dead.

Uncertainty and hesitation on the highway is an invitation to tailgating disaster. Once you've committed yourself to enter traffic, blend swiftly with it and drive as if it were your responsibility to keep it flowing. It is. When all cars on the road move at the same speed, safely spaced, none is likely to get clobbered. A U.S. Bureau of Public Roads study, published in 1964, showed that a third of the cars involved in two-car rear-enders on main rural highways were moving at a speed differential of more than 30 miles an hour. This speed difference is far more dangerous than the actual speed of the car causing the accident.

Being overly cautious is not the only way you can invite trouble for yourself and other drivers. Some others: Open the door of your parked car into traffic. Squat half on the pavement while you change a tire. Mosey along the turnpike at a sightseeing pace. Edge the front of your car a couple of feet onto the highway from the side road, as you wait for space to enter the highway. Get into the fast lane and hold onto it, in spite of the honking horns and blinking lights. Don't bother about the effect of your actions on others. Soon you'll have people guessing and hesitating, and that's pretty sure to bring on a tail-ender.

Shun the bunch.

Tailgaters flock together, like sheep. They ride the highway in clusters of six or eight, 100 feet apart, with a mile of empty road ahead and behind. To defend yourself from them, keep a cushion of space all around. If someone cuts in ahead and fills your cushion, drop back. If somebody rides your tail, increase your speed and leave him, or slow down and wave him past. When you pass another vehicle, *pass*, don't dawdle. In every situation keep thinking of an "out" for whatever may develop.

Check your eyes.

Pennsylvania police told of a driver who had nine rear-end collisions in one year. Called in for examination, he passed the visual-acuity test with a satisfactory 20/30. But he flunked on the test for binocular vision—the ability of the eyes to work together.

Binocular vision is essential in judging speed and distance. In 1957, the American Optometric Association tested 3000 licensed drivers in 25 states and found 22 percent with inadequate binocular vision.

Poor binocular vision is treatable. The Nebraska Safety Engineering and Consulting Service says that acceptable vision can be achieved in about 90 percent of such cases with the aid of proper corrective lenses.

Light up.

A new look at auto lighting might help to reduce the tailgating slaughter. Red is not the most visible color for lights. Moreover, because of common eye defects, many people perceive red lights as being farther away than they really are. Yet all rear warning lights on cars—running, stop and directional—are red.

Why the attachment to red? Why not, as safety engineers have suggested, use different-colored lights to show what a driver is doing—a green running light for instance, to show that he is moving at a constant speed, an amber light to show that he is turning and a bright-orange danger light to show that he has applied his brakes?

Alert the law.

The police admit that tailgating is a major factor in many accidents. But who ever gets a ticket for tailgating, or even a polite warning to alert him to the danger of what he is doing? Within ten miles recently, on a well-traveled throughway, six drivers tailgated me, threatening me and my property. A state patrolman saw one of the threats. He did nothing.

The nation's police wrote three million tickets to restrain speeders in 1964. In New York State alone 2364 drivers had their licenses revoked—and 6746 more had licenses suspended—for repeated speeding violations. But only a relative handful of Americans received tickets in restraint of tailgating. In part, this discrepancy is due to the fact that tailgating is extremely hard to define or prove in court—unless it results in an accident. By then, of course, it is too late.

But it is not too late to try to remedy the situation. Shouldn't we start thinking about the 2000 Americans who will die in rear-end collisions this year? Isn't it time policemen started writing those tickets?

How to Fight
Highway Hypnosis

by Slade Hulbert, with Arlene and Howard Eisenberg

HUMMING through the night along the endless blacktop east of Wendover, Utah, a station wagon suddenly ran off the road and rolled over. The wagon was loaded with blankets and sleeping bags, and the driver was unhurt.

Speeding along a straight and level stretch of U.S. 301 near Whitakers, N.C. at 4:30 a.m., a family driving to a reunion was not so lucky. Their car veered off an embankment and landed upside down in a creek. Eight of the ten passengers, including four small children, drowned.

On a sunny August day, an auto headed west on two-lane State Highway 49 near Lawrenceville, Pa., swerved without warning into the eastbound lane and collided head-on with a camper pickup truck. Both drivers and one passenger died.

These widely scattered accidents had one common denominator: a drowsy driver. The driver of the turned-over station wagon was so sound asleep that he didn't wake up until an emergency wrecker began to right his car. The driver pushing through North Carolina had driven far beyond his endurance. The Pennsylvania driver was evidently drowsy from the afternoon heat.

The problem of the sleepy driver has interested me ever since the warm summer afternoon when, returning home from an exhausting

145

weekend, I fought off sleepiness and finally slammed into a parked car. Since then, as a research psychologist in traffic engineering at the University of California at Los Angeles, I have participated in several studies in which nearly half the drivers interviewed admitted to sleepiness on long trips. A 1973 survey of 1500 drivers conducted by Duke University's department of psychiatry has concluded that "the phenomenon of drowsiness while driving affects nearly two thirds of the driving population." One national study indicates that about two percent of fatal accidents are caused by driver sleepiness.

Although falling asleep at the wheel is not a new phenomenon, it has increased over the years as technology has increased the monotony of driving. Major roads have been engineered to eliminate sharp curves, hills, and bumps, and the automobile is designed to eliminate effort in steering or shifting. The driver sits on a comfortable couch, in a carpeted, soundproofed, temperature-regulated vehicle. Compounding this comfort are the singing of the tires, the steady speed, the drone of the engine, the repetitive pattern of trees and poles.

Often, this monotony leads to the dangerous, trance-like state known as "highway hypnosis." After a tragic train-truck collision in the Southwest, the startled Santa Fe engineer reported that the truck driver had driven into the crossing staring straight ahead, as though totally unaware of the oncoming, whistle-screaming train.

Man's diurnal nature—his custom of working by day and sleeping at night—is also a reason for driver fatigue. Most motorists who are still driving three hours past their normal bedtime will eventually develop an almost irresistible urge to sleep. Another frequent and usually unsuspected villain is carbon monoxide, which not only seeps into cars from faulty exhaust systems, but also feeds through open windows in heavy traffic (where concentrations of carbon monoxide have tested out at seven times safe levels). If concentrations are high enough, unconsciousness can come without warning. But even before symptoms appear (headaches, dizziness, nausea), carbon monoxide can reduce visual acuity and speed of response.

No matter how well rested they may be, some drivers can suddenly fall asleep after as little as 20 minutes at the wheel. They are afflicted with narcolepsy, a potentially dangerous condition which can bring on sleep almost instantly at any time. A Massachusetts driver whom we interviewed described a series of shockingly close calls behind the wheel. Once he awoke with the nose of his car buried in a snowbank. Another time, what woke him was the clash of metal on metal as his car caromed off a guardrail. On a third occasion, he was awakened by the scraping of brush as his car made an unguided S turn across a median and toward traffic speeding in the opposite direction.

One estimate is that there are over 250,000 clear-cut cases of narcolepsy in the United States. But Dr. H. J. Roberts, author of *The Causes, Ecology and Prevention of Traffic Accidents*, believes there may be as many as ten million persons afflicted with varying degrees of the ailment. Most, like the Massachusetts man, are unaware of the condition; they continue to drive, jeopardizing themselves and others.

Although not nearly enough funds are currently being allocated to the development of countermeasures to combat driver fatigue, recent studies at universities and at insurance-company and auto-proving grounds have turned up new and potentially useful knowledge. For example, a variety of highway tests have demonstrated that a driver's behavior changes as he becomes drowsy. While still alert, he is relatively inactive; as he begins to tire, he becomes restless. He squirms in the seat, stretches, scratches, rubs his eyes. He may experience little lapses of attention— as brief as a fraction of a second—of which he is probably unaware. He pays less and less attention to his instrument panel and his rearview and side-view mirrors. He stares fixedly ahead. At this point, the driver's patterns change: he steers less, changes speed irregularly or erratically, weaves back and forth.

Several devices which grab the driver's attention when these changes begin to occur have been patented. Since most are neither fully effective nor practical in terms of cost, highway engineers and traffic-enforcement officers should consider ways to prevent driver sleepiness in the first place.

Roads are a good place to begin. Toll booths at frequent intervals along a turnpike help keep drivers awake—and alive. Other devices for breaking the sight-and-sound rhythm of the road are textures in pavements, noise-making rumble strips, road dividers and raised pavement markers between lanes.

Whatever auto manufacturers and highway engineers accomplish, however, the wise driver knows that the burden of responsibility for safety rests in his own hands. Fortunately, there is much that you as a driver can do to avoid fatigue at the wheel:

• *Plan your trip*. Get an early start, rather than a late one after work. If you must leave straight from work, get some extra sleep the night before. Schedule a food or rest stop every 90 minutes to two hours, and even more often at night. Substitute light snacks at these stops for heavy meals, which can be almost as stupefying as alcohol. Caffeine— in coffee, strong tea and cola drinks—will help stimulate you, but only for a limited time.

• *Check your car carefully*. Before you take off, have a trustworthy mechanic examine your auto's exhaust system. Clean headlights periodically, and both the inside and outside of your windshield. Wear seat and shoulder belts not only for safety but also because they help you avoid the slouching that brings on fatigue.

• *Avoid alcoholic beverages*. Alcohol and drowsiness are frequent accomplices. Avoid smoking, too; it can dim your night vision as much as ten percent. Prescription drugs can also cause drowsiness; before you use any medication when you must drive, check with your physician.

• *Don't drive alone on long trips*. Solo drivers are more sleep-prone than those with someone to talk to. Listening to the radio—especially talk shows, ball games and rock music—can help; but avoid quiet music or droning talk. Whistling and singing can be helpful; also word games that exercise the mind.

• *Exercise*. Prolonged lack of activity is often responsible for driver fatigue. Pulling over at a rest area for exercise—jogging or calisthenics—can provide an effective lift.

• *Break the monotony*. Vary speed levels every 15 minutes or so. Turn on the radio; turn it off. Open the left front window, then close it. And always keep your eyes moving: check instruments, rear-view mirror, road signs, the sides of the road, side-view mirror.

But no matter what you do to ward off weariness, your body will rebel if it is seriously over-extended. At such times nothing—*but nothing*—will really help except getting some rest. So, remember: before you take your next long trip, do more than make sure that your car is in good running condition—make sure that *you* are.

Marijuana and Driving: The Sobering Truth

by Peggy Mann

RECENT STUDIES blow the warning whistle on a little-publicized but nonetheless frightening menace to motorists: the pot smoker driving "high" on the highways. Persuasive evidence is mounting that such drivers often have a distorted sense of space and time, altered peripheral and central vision, and impaired manipulative and coordination skills.

Limited surveys reported by the National Institute on Drug Abuse (NIDA) reveal that 60 to 80 percent of the marijuana users questioned sometimes drive while "intoxicated" on pot. Every day, increasing numbers of stoned drivers are endangering lives—as pot use escalates into what NIDA calls "a national epidemic among young people." (A 1981 countrywide survey showed that one out of every 14 high-school seniors smokes pot *daily*.)

Our nation is both unaware of the marijuana highway crisis and unprepared for it. Many states have inexpensive and legally recognized tests for establishing alcoholic intoxication. However, we have no workable roadside test for marijuana intoxication. (NIDA is funding research on such a test, but it is probably three or four years away from being ready.)

In 39 states, possession of marijuana is still a crime, but enforcement is generally lax—and pot smokers know it. Of the 11 states that have decriminalized marijuana, only Alaska, Colorado, Mississippi, and New

York have thus far enacted a special increased penalty for possession of pot in a vehicle. In all 11 states, many pot-smoking drivers mistakenly believe that decriminalization implies governmental sanction to smoke marijuana—anywhere.

The politicization of pot has helped to obscure the picture. But when emotions and polemics are cleared away, both pro- and anti-decriminalization forces agree that it is dangerous to drive stoned. Even the National Organization for the Reform of Marijuana Laws (NORML), which supports removal of all legal penalties for possession of pot for personal use, "strongly discourages driving while under the influence of marijuana or any other drug, and recognizes the legitimate public interest in prohibiting such conduct."

The "legitimate public interest," however, is *not* being protected. Highway officials nationwide express profound concern. Richard L. Burton, former commissioner of Alaska's Department of Public Safety, has been among the most apprehensive, saying, "The alcohol problem on the highways will soon be only half as serious as marijuana—and that's not because the alcohol problem is going to get any better!" And Lee Dogoloff, former White House adviser on federal drug policy, states: "It is essential that Americans understand the very real hazards of driving while marijuana-intoxicated."

• *How much does marijuana contribute to traffic accidents and fatalities?* Research findings have been remarkably consistent. In 1975, the Boston University Traffic Accident Research Team surveyed 267 drivers deemed "most responsible" for a fatal accident. The investigators estimated that 16 percent of the 267 drivers had been smoking marijuana prior to the fatal accident. Statistically, "marijuana smokers were over-represented in fatal highway accidents," the study concluded.

California's Department of Justice has made the first large-scale study directly relating marijuana to traffic arrests. The study, completed in 1978, covered 46 of the state's 58 counties and examined 1792 blood samples (randomly selected from 19,000 turned in by the California Highway Patrol). The samples were mainly from drivers arrested for traffic accidents, or for impaired driving, or for driving under the influence of drugs. The tests were made with a radioimmunoassay laboratory technique that can analyze blood samples for molecules of THC (tetrahydrocannabinol), the chief mind-altering ingredient of marijuana. Fourteen percent of the 1792 arrested drivers had sufficient THC in their blood to constitute marijuana intoxication.

Victor Reeve, supervisor of the California study, pointed out: "This should be regarded as a conservative figure because, of the drivers arrested, fewer than half agreed to give a blood sample. How many of the remaining drivers were under the influence of marijuana we will never know."

• *How does pot affect driving abilities?* More than 50 studies have been made in the United States since 1970, when standardized grades of so-called "NIDA marijuana" were made available to researchers. Says Herbert Moskowitz, a University of California research psychologist who has probably done the most work on marijuana with simulated driving studies: "The preponderance of evidence indicates that marijuana impairs skills performance and perceptual processes, including vision, attention, and tracking behavior—all important components of driving performance."

Such impairments as tracking performance are significant after two "street joints." Drivers may imagine they are doing a fine job of keeping the car in the correct lane, when in fact they are weaving.

In addition, marijuana can cause: impaired short-term memory function, impaired concentration, impaired ocular motor control and impaired vigilance.

These results are generally obtained in driving-simulator tests—and most people drive *better* under simulated conditions than they drive normally.

However, one test was carried out in *actual* driving conditions by Dr. Harry Klonoff, professor of psychiatry at the University of British Columbia. He chose 64 psychologically stable subjects who had used marijuana before. One third were given a low dosage of one street joint, one third received a high dosage of two joints, the other third received placebos. With dual controls and an observer in each car, all 64 volunteers drove through a closed course with no other traffic. Low-dose subjects showed a 33-percent significant decline in driving skills, while high-dose subjects showed a 55-percent significant decline.

Thirty-eight drivers also covered a 16-mile route from the university campus to the traffic-heavy downtown area, and back again. These 38 were rated by the system used to examine drivers for licensing. Final figures for the road test showed that those on the low dose had a *42-percent decline* in driving skills, while the high-dosage subjects had a *63-percent decline.* Unusual driving behavior, Klonoff reported, included missing traffic lights or stop signs, poor handling of the vehicle in traffic, unawareness of pedestrians and stationary vehicles.

Of 11 behavioral components tested, the three of greatest vulnerability were judgment, caution and concentration—despite the fact that some of the subjects paid special attention to their driving to prove that pot had no impairing effects.

• *How long does marijuana continue to affect driving skills?* Studies in 1972 showed a definite decrease in skills performance five to six hours after intake of a strong social dose of marijuana. Another worrisome factor, reported in 1976 by NIDA, is that a person may attempt to drive without realizing that his functioning is still impaired—even though he or she no longer feels "high."

A 1972 study of driving behavior in a safety-controlled area showed a "marked" decline in driving abilities was still present 5 to 6 hours after intake, a "definite" effect eight to ten hours after intake, and a lingering effect as long as 24 hours later. Another factor: Many chronic pot smokers reported that only a few puffs of "good pot" (with a high THC content) can result in a sudden intense high (if this happens on the highway it can be frightening and dangerous).

• *Do pot users recognize the danger of driving while stoned?* Chronic pot smokers tend to view their driving impairments through rose-colored glasses. Among more than 1000 people arrested for marijuana possession in Minnesota, 25 percent thought pot had no effect on their driving. More than 25 percent thought pot actually improved their coordination. Some enthusiasts *prefer* driving stoned, saying that it becomes less boring. "I get more into my driving" goes the refrain.

Dr. Joseph Davis, the medical examiner in Dade County, Fla., with Arnold W. Klein and Dr. Brian D. Blackbourne surveyed 571 local college and post-graduate students on pot and driving. In every driving category former and infrequent users sharply downgraded their ability to perform while stoned, while chronic pot smokers gave themselves quite good grades. Despite their cheery assessments, 53 percent of the chronic users had been stopped by police for driving under the influence of drugs; 22 percent had three or more violations, compared with 2.3 percent of non-users. Eight percent had had their license revoked, compared to one percent of the non-users.

The alcohol-drunk driver usually finds it hard to hide his condition, if stopped by the police. But the pot-high driver often believes he can "come down" and carry on a seemingly normal conversation with a police officer. This apparent ability to "hide their high" gives many pot smokers confidence that they can drive stoned.

One such self-assured driver, a 30-year-old medical sociologist—a heavy drug user and daily pot smoker for about five years before he swore off drugs—reported smoking a few joints at a friend's house. Then he borrowed his friend's car, certain that he could handle whatever might turn up on the road—including the police. "But," he recalls, "as I drove down one of the busiest streets in the city, the dream-like pleasure I usually felt when driving stoned suddenly burst into a total psychedelic experience. All I could see was a myriad of tiny dancing lights. I was so totally spaced out that I had no awareness of even being *in* a car, much less driving one."

When a traffic light turned red, he didn't notice it, and crashed into a small car. He got out, danced a little jig, walked away and wandered around the city for hours. "I knew something had happened. But I didn't know what."

Around 4 a.m. he remembered, and turned himself in to the police. He learned that he had wrecked his friend's car, and had totally demolished the small car in front of him—which had, in turn, crashed into the sedan in front of it. Remarkably, no one had been seriously injured.

• *What can be done—now*? We need not wait helplessly until scientists come up with a roadside kit for testing THC levels, and states enact laws to deal with marijuana-intoxicated drivers. There are two avenues we can take right away.

First, state legislatures should immediately pass laws imposing a high fine and/or other stiff penalty for possession of marijuana *in a vehicle*—including taxis, buses, trucks, trains, and planes.

Second, we must inaugurate educational programs by governmental agencies, insurance companies, foundations, private groups and, especially, high-school and private-driving instructors. (A friend of mine taking a driving course was offered a joint by an instructor, "to relax.") Coordination of effort will increase the impact of the message: *it's dangerous to drive stoned.*

Brochures should be distributed at toll booths, gas stations, garages. Car users are a captive audience, and "spot warnings" can be tailored to a range of radio programs. The American Automobile Association and National Safety Council could begin a nationwide information campaign.

Unless we move in these directions, warns Robert Willette, who while with NIDA was responsible for developing THC test kits, more and more pot users will be driving high. "We can only hope that growing awareness of the problem," he says, "will prevent a national disaster."

Can You "Talk" to Other Drivers?

by E. D. Fales, Jr.

ONE WINTER, I saw two cars ahead of me spin off an icy bridge in New England. It was raining, and drivers we had met coming our way *knew* that on the bridge the rain had frozen. But they didn't tell us. A friend to whom I mentioned the accident later asked sadly, "But how do you *tell* another driver about a thing like that at 40 miles an hour?"

There is a way—a way in which one driver can communicate with another, alert him to danger, ask his help, say thank you, and otherwise convey the messages that are part of civilized behavior everywhere, it seems, but on the highway. A West Coast driving expert, Harold L. Smith, gave me a demonstration of "driver talk" and of how useful it can be. In a remarkable tour through five states, I watched him "talk" with other drivers at crossroads, in tight passing situations, even in confusing shopping-center parking lots. He talked with headlights, with hand gestures, with the horn—even with the tilt of his head.

Smith, who used to travel over 50,000 miles a year studying driving problems, is the originator of the "Smith System of No-Accident Driving," variations of which have been taught to employe groups in such big corporations as Greyhound Lines, United Parcel and some companies of the Bell System. Firms whose employes drive by Smith's methods have reported a sharp reduction in accidents.

Here are eight "messages" that any alert driver can send:

"I plan to turn left, here!"

Thousands of cars are hit just before making left turns. The reason: the driver doesn't show clearly *where* he plans to turn. In one city, we interviewed a typical victim who had just wrecked both his car and a woman's. "We were on one of those four-lane, undivided suburban roads with traffic moving both ways," he said. "I was in the lane next to the center line; the woman was 200 feet ahead of me. She flashed her left-turn signal. To me it meant, 'I will turn at the next corner.' Instead, she suddenly stopped in mid-block to turn left into a bowling center. I hit her. The next car hit me."

Although the person behind *should* assume that you might turn before the corner, do your best to give a clear message of what you're going to do. To signal such a turn properly, start "drifting" your car gradually toward the center line after you switch on your turn light—*an inch or two at a time*. This drift will be noticed instantly by those behind you. It also uncovers your turn light to drivers several cars back. As the moment of turn approaches, tap your foot brake lightly, to caution any driver who is still following too closely. In the last 100 feet, when you are as close to the center line as you can safely come, your car's unusual position is saying clearly, "I am now ready to turn . . . *here*!"

"I see you . . . and will help."

All of us, on occasion, find ourselves blocking the road for some faster driver who would like to pass. It would relieve the tension if we could let him know, "I see you and will give you passing room as soon as a safe opportunity comes."

To convey this message, says Smith, lift your head once or twice and glance in the rearview mirror. Even a slight tilt of the head is remarkably visible. It says, "I see you." At night, it will also help if you reach up and adjust the mirror. The following driver will see this in the glow of his headlights. Now, as a further courtesy, let your car drift to the right. This makes it easier for the other driver to watch for a safe passing zone and says, "I'll cooperate as soon as I can." Few drivers, noting this, will risk an angry, unwise pass.

There is a chance that the driver behind will interpret your drift to mean, "If you want to pass badly, do it *now*." So, after the first drift,

Smith recommends returning your car to its normal position. The driver behind seems to understand. He drops back a safe distance and waits.

"Danger in your lane! Prepare to stop."

Suppose that you pass a wreck which has occurred in an oncoming-traffic lane. Seconds later, around a curve, you meet cars racing toward the wreck, unaware of danger. A pileup is imminent.

Such situations call for a signal that truck drivers use: rapidly flashing headlights. Truckers began blinking their headlights years ago to warn one another of speed patrols. Today the signal is an alert against any peril: wrecks, sudden ice, children in the road, washouts.

"Danger in my lane! Don't hit me!"

Suppose you see, as I did one day recently in Connecticut, three boulders roll off a truck in front of 60-m.p.h. turnpike traffic. In such a crisis, merely applying brakes is insufficient warning to cars behind you, who may simply rush around you toward disaster. To say, "Emergency!" pump the pedal in a series of fast, hard stabs to *flash* your brake lights. As soon as your car is under control, add a "flag-down" signal by waving your left arm in a wide vertical arc outside the window. Keep your brake lights flashing even after you've stopped.

I have tested this sequence of signals in several emergencies. In the case of the fallen boulders, I saw my "flag-down" wave copied instantly by drivers behind me. Within seconds, the message *Danger!* was relayed to cars far back.

"I am watching out for you."

Horn blasts annoy and even anger young bicyclists. Moreover, the cyclist may look over his shoulder in surprise or fright—and steer directly into your path.

The trouble is, most drivers sound their horns in warning when only four or five car lengths away. The best signal on a quiet street is a light, friendly "beep" sounded eight to ten car lengths (about half a block) away. If necessary, add a second beep, but space the two slightly, to keep a friendly, casual tone. Such early warnings give boys and girls time to adjust their steering calmly.

"Please help me get in line."

All of us find ourselves blocked in side streets or driveways or parking lots by slow-moving traffic crossing our bow. One reason no one wants to let us into the line, Smith says, is that too many of us *demand* to be let in. We point defiantly; we even jam our fenders into the line, then show the palm of our left hand to say, "Stay back there, mister!" We are, Smith says, sending the wrong message.

He showed me the secret of getting into line: Choose one driver in the oncoming line and look at him. And in that look—*ask*! Says Smith: "Try to get eye-to-eye contact. Give him a quick, friendly wave of the hand. And add a big, friendly smile—just in case." With such "talk," Smith says, you rarely have to ask more than two drivers.

"Thanks!"

When a driver makes way for you, thank him. It creates good feeling, makes for safer driving. Many drivers use a half-wave, half-salute. Another signal, used by truck drivers, is two light taps on the horn, sounding almost like *"Thank . . . you."*

"I'm sorry."

At a downtown traffic light in Delaware, a daydreaming driver failed to start when the light turned green. Smith, after a patient wait, nudged his horn. The signal came out harsher than intended. The man glared back at us. Smith said, "Oh-oh, he's mad!"

At the next red traffic light we pulled up alongside that driver. Smith's hand came up in a cheerful little salute. As clearly as if he'd spoken, Smith was saying, "Sorry, friend, those things happen."

The other driver began to smile. And suddenly he was waggling back, a little salute which clearly said, "That's all right, forget it!"

Smith had extended the hand of friendship. And friendship is one of the greatest safety aids of all.

Twelve Suggestions for Safer Driving

Always fasten your seat belt or harness snugly.

Before driving a strange car, reset the seat and mirror, check the "feel" of the brakes and steering. Even with your own, check the mirror each time you drive.

Always look for an "out," a place to steer toward if you get in a jam.

Before moving into another lane, glance back to check the blind spot that your mirror doesn't show.

Keep the car moving at a reasonable speed, or get it off the road—completely and then some.

Anticipate stops and slowdowns; don't wait until you're out of adequate space.

In slowing, pump your brakes to flash your taillights.

When passing, wait before cutting back until you can see the passed car in your mirror.

On multi-lane roads, remember that the right-hand lane is likely to be more slippery than the passing lane, especially when wet, because of wear and oil-spatter.

If your windshield is dirty, so are your headlights; be sure to clean them or get them cleaned when you stop for gas.

You pass the peak of your driving efficiency between your fifth and sixth hours at the wheel; near the end of their driving day, the real pros always slow down and take it easy, or they take rest breaks during the day.

Never hesitate to yield the right of way, especially if the other driver is at fault. The best place for a faulty driver is out of your way.

—Changing Times
The Kiplinger Magazine.

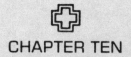

CHAPTER TEN

DRIVING
IN HAZARDOUS CONDITIONS

Ten Tips
for Winter Driving

by Col. Gilbert R. Carrel *as told to* Curtis W. Casewit

A FEBRUARY blizzard was raging when I headed south from Denver on a drive I'll never forget. Snow and ice covered the highways; it was even snowing in Louisiana, my destination. All through the Gulf States, I saw motorists in trouble. Yet I had no difficulty in reaching New Orleans.

How did I make it? Simple. My car was equipped for winter. After all, I live in the state that calls itself "The Top of the Nation," and over the years I've learned a few tricks about winter driving. Let me share some pointers with you.

• First, take pains to see that your car is ready for winter. Be sure the motor is tuned up, the brakes function properly, the battery is good, and the headlights and taillights are working. In your trunk, keep a shovel, a bag of sand and chains in case you encounter deep snow.

I've found that motorists sometimes neglect minor items such as perfect windshield wipers. They're excellent life insurance. Not long ago we investigated a crash in eastern Colorado. Two cars had collided head-on during a bad snowfall because one of the drivers had failed to buy new wiper-blades. He wanted to save four dollars—instead he spent thousands in hospital bills.

Clean windshields—front and back—are absolutely essential for bad-weather driving. That's why I recommend a small brush to wipe

163

off snow, plus a scraper to remove ice from the entire window. Also, you may want to consider snow blades.

• On packed snow and ice, your tires are, of course, the most important part of your car. Slick tires are like sleds—you just can't stop them. One December, I rushed to the scene of a major accident involving four cars. Eight persons died because *one* car had bald tires.

Most motorists find snow tires a wise investment. Tires with steel studs (illegal in some states) also do an excellent job on ice. But in blizzard conditions, *nothing* can match chains.

To prove that point, the National Safety Council and the American Automobile Association ran an experiment. They let a car cross a patch of ice at 20 m.p.h. On regular tires, the car needed 149 feet to stop. The same car, equipped with rear-wheel chains, stopped in 75 feet.

• Next to your tires, brakes are the most important element in combating icy roads. To test braking power on a wintry road, see how your brakes act at about 20 m.p.h. When you have to stop on snow, pump your brakes, using them lightly and *intermittently*, thus reducing the chance of a skid. With disc brakes, the pumping action should be slower.

Skidding, the main winter-driving problem, produces a bone-chilling sensation. What should you do? Keep calm; stay off the brakes; ease off the accelerator; don't release the wheel. *Steer in the direction that you want the front end of the car to go*. Don't oversteer, and you will be all right. A good rule of thumb is this: If you expect icy conditions, drive slowly, turn slowly, brake before you hit ice patches, and use restraint and steadiness in your steering. It's easier to recover at a slow pace.

• When visibility nears zero, park awhile, but be sure that the exhaust pipe does not get clogged with snow. Try to wait until weather improves. Keep your heater going and a window open (fresh air is much better than carbon monoxide). Stay a sensible distance from the next parked car. If you get too close, and the other car's motor is running, *your* heater can draw in the fumes.

Here are some other suggestions:

• Keep your tank filled with gas. The fuller the tank, the less condensation of water, and the less chance of a fuel-line freeze-up.

• When driving downhill or around curves, use lower gears.

• If you must drive in bad weather, always use the lower headlight beams (but never parking lights). The upper beams will reflect off fog and snow, and blind you.

• Not all rental cars come with chains or snow tires. Insist on these items or go to another agency.

• Stuck in a snowdrift? Clear away as much snow from around the tires as possible. Spread a little sand or ashes under the rear tires, or use a traction mat. Then gently rock the car back and forth, shifting from forward to reverse. A little rocking will free you.

• Finally, remember that poor winter-driving conditions don't cause accidents—poor drivers do!

How to Drive in Fog

Crashes in New York, Illinois, Georgia, Florida and elsewhere have involved 10, 20, even 50 cars and trucks. One in California involved 234. The horror of chain collisions is heightened by the fact that many of the trucks, running full tilt to maintain schedules, carry flammables or explosives. Until we find better ways of monitoring fog on super-highways, and of conveying traffic through it, each driver is on his own. Some suggestions:

• Watch out for sudden patches of fog when approaching rivers, bridges, swamps, coastal areas—especially during the very early morning hours. Be wary of river-valley roads in autumn, hilltop roads in winter.

• In any fog, day or night, use your headlights, not parking lights, so other drivers will see you. High beams create too much glare, yet in night fog it is not safe to run on low beams only. So flick your beams repeatedly to high to reveal reflectorized danger objects that simply can't be seen with low beams. Before entering patches of fog, flash your brake warning lights to let other drivers know you're slowing down.

• Turn on your windshield wipers, washer and defroster if any film forms. Some of the "fog" may simply be mist on the glass.

• As fog cuts visibility, slow down and increase the cushion between you and traffic ahead. When visibility drops to three to five car lengths, get off the road to a safe place and light your hazard flasher. Above all, don't be lured into one of those 20- and 30-car chains that go whistling through fog following the taillights of the car ahead.

• In case of accident, get everyone out of your car *instantly*. Tell them to run at right angles to the road, as far as possible from the road. If you stay behind to help, try to stay on the shoulder, and keep an ear cocked for the sound of approaching vehicles.

• Remember that the first rule of superhighway driving in fog is: don't, if you can possibly avoid it.

—*Popular Mechanics*

Pills
Drivers Shouldn't Take

by Evan McLeod Wylie

A NEW JERSEY housewife, driving with her two children, swung into fast-moving turnpike traffic. Then suddenly, she recalls, "the road seemed to billow up and down. Speeding cars and trucks were all around me, but I couldn't make my eyes focus. A huge bus let out a terrific blast on its horn. I had veered out of my lane, and the bus had missed us by inches. Only by gripping the steering wheel with all my might was I able to guide the car into a gas station and stop."

A few hours earlier, this young mother had swallowed a sedative prescribed by her physician. The side effects of the drug had almost caused a tragic accident.

Increasingly, such drivers, unaware of possible side effects of seemingly harmless medication, are causing medical authorities grave concern. A Texas psychiatrist became aware of an alarming number of auto accidents befalling patients for whom he had prescribed moderate to strong doses of an anxiety-reducing drug. Reviewing a series of such reports, the doctor discovered that in a 90-day period, of 68 patients taking the drug, ten were involved in minor and six in major accidents—a rate ten times higher than would have been predicted for a normal cross section of population.

Drugs ranging from antihistamines to tranquilizers may slow a driver's reaction time and impair his performance, according to Drs. Carlos

Perry and Alan Morgenstern in the *Journal of the American Medical Association*. Another professional publication, the *Medical Letter*, reported to its doctor-subscribers that dozens of drugs affect the central nervous system in ways that can impair driving ability. It noted that more than 50 percent of the drug advertisements in a leading medical journal contained warnings of side effects such as drowsiness, visual disturbances and vertigo.

Many pain-killing drugs wear off quickly, but some side effects can linger up to 48 hours. One physician suggests that a patient might not regain his full reflex activity or be capable of exerting his best judgment for up to two days. And sleeping pills containing barbiturates induce hypnotic effects up to 14 hours so that the drug taken the night before may still be at work when you drive to the office in the morning.

One frequently prescribed tranquilizer carries precautions which should bar its use by anyone who drives. The manufacturer states: "As is true of most preparations containing central nervous system-acting drugs, patients receiving this drug should be cautioned against engaging in hazardous occupations requiring complete mental alertness such as operating machinery or driving a motor vehicle." Hundreds of users fail to observe this warning.

Many people, unmindful of the risk involved, use several drugs at the same time. They may, for example, take a tranquilizer in the morning, swallow antihistamines or aspirin or cough syrup for a cold during the day, and then, after work, have a cocktail. "Such practices," commented Drs. Perry and Morgenstern, "are especially dangerous for motorists, because the multiple or antagonistic action of these combinations increases the difficulty of predicting the effects."

Another scientist observes, "Many people are dosing themselves with combinations that we wouldn't dare try in a laboratory, let alone behind the wheel of a car."

The most insidious hazard for people who take drugs and drive lies in what pharmacologists call the "escalating" or "potentiating" reaction when an alcoholic beverage collides with a drug. The alcohol and the drug react together on the central nervous system with devastating effect. For example, a tranquilizing pill combined with only a slight amount of alcohol becomes a sleeping pill. Similarly, a sleeping pill of the barbiturate type can, when combined with alcohol, become a poison capable of causing dizziness, blackout, even death. Since the effects vary enormously from person to person, the amount of alcohol or of drug consumed need not be great. After the recent sudden death of a famous writer, the medical examiner said, "It could have been simply one extra pill."

Some doctors consider one tranquilizing pill equal to one drink. For many persons it may be far more potent. One physician asserts that one pill plus one drink may equal four drinks.

Dr. Robert Forney, of the Indiana University School of Medicine, points out that the person who customarily uses alcohol in acceptable social amounts doesn't realize, when required by illness to take drugs, that he must then carefully limit his drinks if he drives.

By standard practice, prescription drugs simply carry a label with directions typed up by the druggist. On it are the number of the prescription, the date, the doctor's name and a brief directive, such as *"One capsule every six hours."* Seldom is there any mention of driving.

Dr. Seward E. Miller, of the University of California at Los Angeles, advocates that certain prescription drugs be placed in containers labeled with a warning symbol—such as a wheel combined with crossbones. Dr. Miller would also like to see a strengthening of the cautionary words on over-the-counter drugs. Warnings such as *"If drowsiness occurs, do not drive"* are usually in fine print. "By the time the drowsiness has occurred," Dr. Miller comments, "it may be too late for anything but a tow truck and an ambulance."

Are doctors doing all they can to warn patients that drugs may decrease driving skill?

According to a spokesman for the American Medical Association, "When a physician is dealing with any person over 16, he should be aware that that person is probably a driver. We want doctors to be more wary of drugs and possible driving impairment. We hope that physicians are taking all precautions in informing patients about side effects when prescribing drugs." To resolve this situation, the AMA has routinely carried warnings about drugs and driving in a widely circulated manual.

Meanwhile you can help your physician guard you against automobile accidents and possible death by asking him about the medicine he prescribes for you, and whether it will affect your driving. Tell him how much you drive, how far, in what kind of traffic. The more he knows, the better he can advise and prescribe for you, and the less danger from drugs you will run.

How to Drive
Out of Trouble

by Robert S. Strother

MRS. Brenda Elliott, a Milford, Mich. secretary, was driving home after a rain squall last summer when she crested a hill and found a fallen tree across her path. "If that had happened two months earlier," Mrs. Elliott said, "I'd have jammed on the brakes, locked the wheels and skidded into a crash. But I was lucky. Some friends had persuaded me to take an advanced driver-education course not long before, and I knew what to do. I could almost hear my instructor saying, 'Hang in there and steer your way out of trouble!' That's exactly what I did and—who knows?—it may have saved my life."

Mrs. Elliott is one of the fortunate thousands who have learned the value of a safety movement called "postgraduate driver education." Ranging from a simple review of the basics to strenuous training in dealing with road crises, these courses are helping to reduce the heavy toll of U.S. motor-vehicle accidents—17.9 million of them in 1980 alone. National Safety Council figures show that 73 percent of these accidents were caused by poor driving, with alcohol a factor in at least half.

Although probably half the licensed drivers in the United States received basic training in high-school driving courses, such instruction touched only the rudiments. Now traffic authorities have begun to realize that the highway death toll remains high partly because people have forgotten what they learned, and still more because they were never taught what to do in emergencies. And there wasn't anywhere to go for help.

Now that situation is beginning to change.

The most promising postgraduate driving programs to date have grown out of the special training auto companies give their test drivers. General Motors, for example, conducted research to identify the causes of most accidents and to find techniques to deal with them. The advanced driver-education course they then developed was first demonstrated to traffic-safety officials in 1969 at GM's big proving ground in Milford, Mich. Now their instructor-training workshop, under Richard A. "Doc" Whitworth, is organizing courses in university safety centers where high-school driving instructors are trained. After four hours of chalk talks and film presentations, interspersed with 12 hours on the driving course, they will be qualified to pass their new skills along to pupils. Within a few years, 20 centers had adopted the GM program, built the necessary driving facility and were teaching hundreds of driving instructors how to cope with emergencies.

In 1973, I took the training at Appalachian State University's new safety center in Boone, N.C., and discovered that I had a lot to learn about what to do in emergency traffic situations.

Learning to control a skid is the "hairiest" exercise in the program. The four training cars are standard models in most ways, but the skid car has a sneaky little button which lets the instructor lock the rear wheels suddenly. As I was crossing the wet skid pad at 20 m.p.h., the rear of the car abruptly skidded left. I counter-steered left and felt the car straightening up nicely. But it began skidding right. A counter-steer in that direction brought the rear end back again, but then it went left as before. It took me three or four embarrassing swoops before I got the beast tamed. My instructor explained: "What this teaches is not to relax after you've corrected the first skid. You've got to be ready to correct the counter-slide if you don't catch it all the first time."

Proper hand position—a firm grip at nine and three o'clock on the wheel—and alertness are stressed in each of the emergency maneuvers taught in the advanced course. In many situations it is smarter to dodge than to brake. In learning evasive action, the trainee dashes down a lane at 35 m.p.h. Sixty feet from a rubber pylon cone barrier, his instructor barks "left" or "right," and the student must swerve without knocking down any cones. A few runs, a lot of work setting cones back in place, and I began to get the knack.

Another exercise requires weaving in and out of a single line of cones at 40 m.p.h. After you achieve reasonable competence, the instructor provides a final ordeal. He lets some air out of a couple of tires and has you run the route again. Improper pressures make your car wander obstinately all over the lot. That, you are told, is the unsuspected cause of many accidents. Your best bet is to buy a tire gauge and check pressures once a week yourself.

All the schools work to remedy the bad habits that creep into almost everybody's driving: riding the brake, failure to pass decisively, cutting curves too close, tailgating, failure to signal lane changes, failure to make constant use of rear-vision mirrors and, above all, failure to anticipate and take defensive action when trouble starts brewing in the traffic situation.

There is no doubt that such training helps reduce both the number and the severity of accidents. The Alabama Safety Center at the University of Montevallo, for instance, was established in 1970 when Alabama, stung by being rated flat last in traffic safety among the 50 states, used $350,000 of its highway-safety funds for driver education. Doc Whitworth and his team trained the first five Montevallo instructors, and their influence has been felt all over the southeastern states. Fatal accidents in Montevallo's home county of Shelby were cut by more than half, and Alabama's traffic-fatality rate dropped from 6.4 per 100 million miles in 1970 to 3.2 in 1980.

In Oakland County, Mich., the sheriff's department asked GM in 1969 to train some of their patrolmen for emergencies. Thirty officers were chosen, and 30 others who matched them were kept out for comparison. After two years, the trained group had been in five accidents, with no injuries and no time or wages lost. Damage to their vehicles was $1446.50. The untrained group had ten accidents, 87 days of work and $3500 in wages lost, and $11,347 in vehicle damage, plus the cost of three cars demolished. Thus the costs of the untrained group due to accidents were almost 20 times those of the trained group.

"We are training all our men now," says Jerry Girard, safety officer for the sheriff's department. "And I'd like to see emergency handling know-how taught every motorist before he gets a license."

No such requirement is likely in the near future, since the 20 existing university centers are fully occupied teaching educators and police, and few commercial schools are equipped to offer such training. Meanwhile, can the average motorist improve his performance just by reading an article like this?

"Of course he can," Doc Whitworth says. "He will have a much better idea of what he should and should not do in a crisis."

Here, for instance, are rules I learned from experts that can help in common driving emergencies:

1. *An obstacle suddenly appears ahead.* Take your foot off the gas and glance quickly ahead and in your mirror. Simultaneously, apply your brake in a series of "spurts," letting off pressure almost as soon as applied in order to avoid wheel lockup. If there's no opposing traffic, swerve around the obstacle left or right, but preferably to the right. If you're on a two-lane road with cars coming, swerve out onto the right shoulder.

2. *You go off the pavement.* If you are forced or have slipped off onto a soft shoulder and the pavement's edge is a few inches high, reduce speed to gain control of your car and return to the pavement. If, however, you are approaching an obstacle such as a mailbox and are forced to return to the road at highway speed, first slow down, straddle the edge of the pavement, and steer sharply left back up onto the road. But remember to return the steering wheel to the straight-ahead position the *instant* the right front wheel hits the edge of the pavement, so you don't shoot into another lane.

3. *You start to skid.* Turn your wheels in the direction you want the front end of the car to go, and let up on the gas without touching the brakes. But, as you bring your car out of the skid, be ready to steer into the *opposite* direction if a counter-skid occurs—as it often does.

4. *You have a blowout.* Especially if you have been traveling fast, grip the wheel hard, using the proper position (hands at nine and three o'clock), and steer to maintain your lane position. Allow the car to slow down before you touch the brake, and then use it very gently. If traffic permits, steer off to the side of the road once you have nearly stopped.

5. *You run into a hard rain flurry.* At high speed in a really bad downpour, your tires can't squeeze the water away fast enough, and they may, especially if under-inflated or worn, not be in contact with the pavement at all. You may, in other words, be hydroplaning and you may not realize you have no traction until you jam on the brakes. Slow down *before* you lose control—to 35 m.p.h. or less.

6. *Your engine conks out coasting down a hill.* Your power brakes and steering no longer have power assistance. So put the emergency brake full on. Then push the brake pedal all the way down to the floor and steer hard. You still have brakes and steering, but it will take a lot more strength than usual to use them.

7. *A car comes at you head on.* Brake in a controlled manner and swerve to the right. Blow your horn, too, because the other driver may be dozing. Turn right off the road if necessary. Better to end in a ditch than in a head-on collision.

"Above all," GM's Whitworth says, "don't panic in an accident, and never give up! In most situations you can steer yourself out of trouble even after the accident sequence begins."

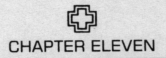

CHAPTER ELEVEN

DANGER
ON TWO WHEELS

Safety-First
for Cyclists

by Thomas R. Brooks

GARY BURNS, a wiry, towheaded ten-year-old, rode his new three-speed bicycle to school each day. One morning he ran a stop sign, and never did see the speeding caterer's truck. Thrown ten feet by the crash, Gary was dead-on-arrival at the hospital.

Gary was one of 1150 deaths in 1973 resulting from roughly 40,000 automobile/bicycle collisions, a scary toll that jumped 98 percent in ten years. In addition, safety authorities estimate that each year over a million cyclists are injured seriously enough to require professional medical treatment.

One reason for the high number of accidents is that we have had a bicycling boom, set off by a broadening interest in improving our health as well as our environment, and by the energy crisis. Sales of new bicycles hit a 15.3-million high in 1973, double the number sold in 1970.

Over 100 million Americans use bicycles to go to and from work, for shopping, exercise and sheer riding pleasure. "We think of cycling as a sport," says John Auerbach, manager of the Cycle Parts and Accessories Association. "But once you are out on the street, you are doing more than exercising; you are operating a vehicle in traffic." And the bicycle is a vulnerable vehicle, indeed, in a world of whizzing automobiles, potholed streets, soft shoulders and angry dogs.

Cycling accidents head the list of product-related injuries drawn up recently by the U.S. Consumer Product Safety Commission. But the stress belongs on *related*, for analysis shows that accidents due specifically to faulty construction are not as frequent as those caused by improper maintenance, and such factors as falls, bumps, double-riding, stunting, and collisions with cars.

One clear way to reduce the number of auto/bike accidents is to separate the two vehicles as some communities have. Bike paths in Sausalito, Calif., are isolated from both automotive and pedestrian traffic by a narrow greensward. Boulder, Colo., constructed an asphalt bike path on the urban floodplain of a local creek, providing a safe bike corridor through the town's business section. Tiburon, Calif., converted an abandoned railroad right-of-way into a car-free bike path.

Still, it is not feasible, or economically possible, to build an entirely separate network of bike paths to parallel the nation's 3.9 million road miles, and thus it is clear that cyclists and motorists will continue to share highway space. How can they do so in greater safety?

Of primary importance is education for all concerned. Motorists *must* realize that bicyclists have a right to their fair share of roadway. Advises Paul St. Mauro, head of the traffic-safety department of the North Jersey Automobile Club: "When you are driving a car and see a cyclist, be wary. Make sure the road ahead is clear before you pass, and never pass on a curve. Assume that the cyclist may do the wrong thing at any time. Give yourself time to brake or veer."

For their part, far too many bicyclists—both young and old—have never received formal training. To help get the safety message across, we need "show and do" bike-proficiency courses. In Nassau County, New York, 10,000 grade-school youngsters each year get on-the-road instruction at sessions in a two-acre "safety village" where they operate electric cars and bicycles.

Each year, the El Cajon, Calif., police department selects 12 high-school honor students to serve as clerks and justices on a special bicycle court that meets Saturdays at the municipal courthouse. More than 14,000 children between the ages of 9 and 17 have appeared as offenders since the court was established in 1965—and only two bicycle fatalities have been recorded in that time. "The whole idea," says one of the honor students, "is to make kids understand what they do wrong."

Here is what you can do to make cycling safe for your family:

• Don't buy an over-size model, expecting your youngster to "grow into it." (Bicycles that are too big or small, as one safety study wryly put it, are "over-represented in collisions with automobiles.") You should be able to straddle the bike frame with both feet on the ground and the horizontal bar just touching your crotch. The seat is at the proper height when the sitting rider's leg is almost fully extended with the ball of the foot on a pedal in its lowest position.

• Make certain that the bike's equipment is appropriate for your child's age. Youngsters under ten do not have the reach or strength to operate hand brakes safely; they need coaster brakes. "High-rise" handlebars, which force a small child to steer with elbows at chin-level, and the long, narrow "banana" seats, which invite additional passengers, are major contributors to instability—and may cause additional accidents. (A good rule is: one person, one bike.) All bikes should have a loud horn or bell.

• In too many bike/car accidents, either the motorist did not see the cyclist or the cyclist did not see the motorist. Brightly colored clothing boosts visibility. International orange is good, and can be found in a light-reflective cloth used in jackets and gloves made for cyclists. If you cycle at night, lights are *essential*. Rear lights are especially important and ought to be visible from 500 feet away. The taillight should be visible from the rear and both sides. Reflectors are a safety backup to lights; a three-inch diameter is a good size. Reflector tape on cycling shoes, fenders, belts, frame, pedals and handlebars also increases visibility.

• Perform routine maintenance regularly: tighten spokes, bolts and screws, adjust chain and brakes, add air to the tires. Take your bike to a bike shop for checkups. Key bearings ought to be disassembled, cleaned and repacked every 500 miles. The chain should be removed, cleaned and lubricated twice a year.

Of course, safe equipment can't by itself guarantee safe riding. To help you to wheel and deal while actually in traffic, the National Safety Council offers these suggestions:

• Obey all applicable traffic regulations, signs, signals and markings. Cyclists are subject to the same rules as motorists. It is your responsibility to know, and abide by, state and local traffic laws. For example, most states require you to ride single file. Most also require a headlight, taillight or red rear reflectors for night cycling. Others require reflective pedals, additional side reflectors or other reflective material.

• Keep right: *ride with traffic, not against it*. Keep close to the right, watching out for drain grates, soft shoulders, loose sand, or gravel— and especially for car doors opening and for cars pulling into traffic.

• Since most accidents happen at intersections, be extremely careful there, especially when making a left turn. If traffic is heavy, walk your bike with pedestrian traffic.

• Use hand signals to indicate turning or stopping.

• Ride defensively. Leave enough room between yourself and the car in front of you to give you time to take defensive action.

Remember: Good cycling is safe cycling—and enjoy yourself.

✚

Moped Madness

by Daphne Hurford

THE TRADITIONAL American response to personal transportation has been the larger, flashier and faster the better. But, battered by the economic crunch, the energy crunch and the air-quality crunch, Americans are beginning to question the way they get around.

Enter the moped. More than a bicycle, less than a motorcycle, mopeds suddenly seem to be an answer. U.S. sales jumped from 25,000 in 1975 to an estimated 150,000 in 1977, and in four more years total sales had reached over a million.

For all the moped pluses—cost (between $450 and $1000), fuel economy (a gallon of gas every 100 to 200 miles) and few pollutants ($\frac{1}{25}$ the amount of a standard automobile)—the overriding reason they are so popular is that they are so much fun.

A moped is a two-wheeled vehicle that, as its name implies, uses both a motor and a pedal-operated chain drive for power. The motor is small, which means it occasionally needs help getting up hills. That (and starting the machine) is where the pedals come in; in such situations, the rider provides the extra boost in power to get, or keep, the thing going.

Approximately 30 models of mopeds were sold in the United States in 1978. The two states with the greatest number of mopeds were New Jersey and California. California also had the most stringent exhaust-emission-control laws in the land. Mopeds were made legal for street use in California (nowhere in America are they permitted on limited-access highways) on January 1, 1976, and sales grew quickly.

In Massachusetts, New York, Ohio and Florida, too, moped madness reached epidemic proportions. As of November 1, 1977, there were an estimated 18,000 mopeds in the Sunshine State. Middle-aged vacationers were two-wheeling all over southern Florida.

As mopeds become more popular, concern mounts over reckless use of the vehicles. There have been injuries and some fatalities, but no one knows the extent of moped accidents because the statistics usually are not separated from those for motorcycles or bicycles.

Moped madness caught not only American manufacturers unaware but the safety establishment as well. Originally, the U.S. government classified mopeds with motorcycles. That meant the same safety standards regarding brakes, tires, lights and controls applied to mopeds with a top speed of 30 m.p.h. as to a motorcycle capable of triple that performance. In October 1974, following a petition by three French moped manufacturers, the National Highway Traffic Safety Administration re-classified mopeds as a subcategory of motorcycles, and created new and more appropriate safety standards. Hand brakes were permitted, turn signals no longer were necessary and taillight candlepower requirements were reduced.

In January 1975, the three French manufacturers, along with other importers, distributors and dealers, formed the Motorized Bicycle Association, now called the Moped Association of America. One of the MAA's major functions has been to encourage individual states to classify mopeds separately from motorcycles so that, for example, riders don't have to wear helmets or carry liability insurance. By the end of 1977, 32 states and the District of Columbia had enacted laws that classified mopeds as something between a bicycle and a motorcycle, with Maine being one of the latest. And as Maine goes....

Well, sort of. The welter of conflicting legislation and regulation concerning mopeds is still cause for confusion. While all the states that permit moped use restrict the machines to two horsepower or less and a small 50-cubic-centimeter engine, most states require a driver's license; in others you need only be 14 and have a permit. Some places have *no* license, registration or insurance requirements.

Confusion notwithstanding, the moped market continues to expand. The first flurry of sales was to students looking for inexpensive, easy-to-park transportation for short distances. Now the majority of buyers seem to be in the 25-to-50 age group; commuters are riding mopeds to train and bus stations; suburbanites are mopedaling to the tennis courts and the market; city dwellers ride them to and from work.

Such buyers are split between those seeking practicality and those simply delighted with a new form of recreation. A group of women in affluent Walnut Creek, Calif., represent the fun-loving element. Wearing T-shirts emblazoned with THE MOPED MAMAS, the women, ages 30 to 65, meet Wednesdays for group runs on their mopeds.

In addition to practicality and pleasure, mopeds have another lure: they are only slightly more complicated than a bobby pin. The models have two-cycle engines, similar to an outboard motor. None have transmissions that demand the coordination of hand and foot required by motorcycles. Instead, they come with "automatic transmissions" (actually clutches with a lot of slippage), and the drum brakes are controlled by handlebar-mounted levers. The least expensive mopeds generally rely only on their skinny wheels to absorb road shocks, which can make them skittish on ripply road surfaces, but as the price goes up, so do suspension sophistication and, as a result, ride control and comfort.

If the moped's sudden success if based largely on its simplicity—anyone who has taken the training wheels off his two-wheeler can master the motorized version almost instantly—so are the potential problems.

Sgt. Lance Erickson of the California highway patrol says, "In almost all collisions the operator of a moped ends up in the hospital. The injury factor is very high." Bruno Porrati, former president of Vespa of America, emphasizes, "A moped is not a toy. It must not be treated as one." And a Florida motorcycle shop owner says, "It's not a bicycle. It has a motor that will go fast enough to get you in trouble, but not fast enough to get you out."

PART FOUR
FIRST AID

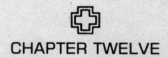

CHAPTER TWELVE

BE PREPARED

The Tag
That Can Save
Your Life

by Richard Dunlop

THE DRIVER slouched over the wheel as the auto wove from one curb to the other, then twisted to a stop at right angles to traffic. Two police officers patrolling Chicago's South Side in a squad car saw the mishap and pulled up beside the motorist, who, flushed and glassy-eyed, was fumbling at the door handle of his car.

Everything seemed to indicate that the driver was drunk, so he was taken to the police station and given an alcohol test. But the test revealed that he had *not* been drinking. By then he had become unconscious. When he was rushed to a hospital, doctors pronounced him a diabetic in insulin shock, a critical condition which resembles drunkenness so closely that it can fool experts.

Such cases are not rare. Millions of Americans have hidden medical problems and dangerous allergies about which first-aiders should know before giving them emergency treatment. Incorrect emergency treatment of such people has long worried police, firemen, first-aid teams and doctors. They know that every year some of the nation's 10.7 million diabetics are locked up as drunks, instead of getting the medical care they need. In emergencies, people are given injections or pills containing penicillin, aspirin, codeine, novocaine or sulfa. If they are allergic to these drugs, the treatment may do more harm than good. Victims of cerebral palsy, heart trouble and epilepsy sometimes receive the wrong first aid.

189

In 1962, the nation's doctors, working through the American Medical Association, announced a new universal symbol which at a glance tells first-aid workers that its wearer has a condition requiring special attention. Hexagonal in shape, it may be displayed on a wristlet, anklet, medallion or card.

The alerting symbol is designed to resemble a stop sign—a familiar shape to most Americans—so that it will say "Stop" to those who see it. Within the outline is the star that is the medical symbol for life, similar to the asterisk which refers one elsewhere for more information—in this case, to a purse, billfold or pocket. Superimposed on the star is a staff with a snake entwined about it—the staff of Aesculapius, the hallowed insigne of the medical profession. Usually, the condition requiring urgent attention can also be imprinted.

Already more than 100,000 Americans are wearing an alerting emblem called Medic-Alert, devised in 1953 by Dr. Marion C. Collins, a Turlock, Calif., general practitioner. Medic-Alert's story started when Dr. Collins' daughter Linda, then 14, cut a finger on a rifle trigger at a target range. At the hospital a doctor, preparing to give her a shot of tetanus antitoxin, made the routine scratch test with one drop of the serum. Suddenly the girl fell to the floor, writhing in convulsions. The serum had triggered a terrifying allergic reaction known as anaphylaxis. For three days Linda gasped for breath in an oxygen tent before she was out of danger.

Dr. Collins wondered how he could protect Linda from a second such experience. He knew that if she were ever given a shot of tetanus antitoxin she would die. As long as Linda stayed in Turlock, a San Joaquin Valley town of 10,000 people, such a likelihood was remote because the whole town had heard of her brush with death. But as Linda prepared to go away to college the problem became acute. The family sat down and puzzled out the answer. Linda would wear a silver bracelet engraved with the warning, "Allergic to Tetanus Antitoxin." On the bracelet, Dr. Collins put the staff of Aesculapius and the words "Medic-Alert" in bright red.

His daughter was now protected, but what about the other Americans—an average of one in every family—who should carry emergency medical identification? The nation's 2,300,000 epileptics, as well as its diabetics, can easily be mistaken for drunk when they are ill. One in every 10,000 males is a hemophiliac who may bleed to death after an injury, if not treated appropriately. Many of our 41 million cardiovascular patients take anticoagulants which must be counteracted by other drugs to prevent excessive bleeding in an accident. Other heart patients are vulnerable to common anesthetics, stimulants and sedatives.

A large number of our 31.6 million arthritis sufferers take corticosteroid drugs, such as prednisone. After shock or injury, complications can be serious or fatal unless these persons are given one of these drugs.

Dr. Collins established the Medic-Alert Foundation to provide protective wristlets for persons throughout the United States; later the protection was extended to other countries. Medic-Alert members not only received their emblems of stainless steel or silver, but their health histories were filed at Turlock, together with the addresses of each member's physician and nearest relative. In an emergency, a doctor or other authorized person could phone collect to Turlock and be given information vital to the Medic-Alert Foundation member's treatment.

Other organizations with the altruistic purpose of benefiting people with health problems were formed, but such organizations could grow only as fast as limited personnel and funds permitted. Pressure mounted for a national approach to the problem. In April 1961, representatives of the nation's major medical and health organizations met in Chicago at the invitation of the American Medical Association. A year later, the proposals of the committee were accepted by the AMA.

"You are an individual—you are unique," the AMA advised Americans. "Possibly you are one who has a medical problem so critical that you must be *sure* it is known to those who help you in an emergency. If so, a signal device should be worn around your neck, wrist or ankle in such a way that it can be present at all times—even in swimming.

"This device should be made of durable material, and it should be fastened to the person wearing it with a strong non-elastic cord or chain, so designed that it does not become an accident hazard in itself."

The AMA urged Americans with health problems that could be troublesome in an emergency to ask their doctor if they should wear a signal device. At the same time, the AMA asked these Americans to carry a medical identification card such as the one designed for the country's doctors. The card contained space for the individual to list his present medical problems, the medicines he took regularly, his dangerous allergies and other information that would help ensure proper care in an emergency. After each entry the individual wrote the date on which he made the entry. Then he showed his card to his doctor to be sure it was accurate in all details.

Did the new universal symbol supersede the existing symbols of established programs? No. It was intended to complement them.

In 1982, the National Safety Council in Chicago announced that it had developed a new medical information card. The wallet-size card carries vital medical data on a strip of microfilm and has a built-in lens. In an emergency, a rescuer need only bend the plastic card to bring the lens and microfilm together to read the accident victim's medical history.

A person who does not speak English should wear a signal device so that it can speak for him in case of trouble. The deaf and mute need the protection of a signal device. So do people who wear contact lenses. (If left on an unconscious accident victim for 24 hours or more, such lenses could damage the cornea of the eye and impair vision or cause severe eye damage. Alcoholics who take Antabuse need protection; they will become violently ill if they are given even a small swallow of liquor or drugs dissolved in alcohol.

There are, in fact, some 200 conditions which require that a person carry emergency medical identification to ensure correct first aid—200 reasons why identifying tags will save lives.

Are You Accident-Prone?

by Stanley L. Englebardt

• In Atlanta, a young housewife listened silently as her husband berated her for running up a big department-store bill. Later, she got into the family car and promptly backed into a tree. Result: a severe whiplash injury and $500 worth of auto damage.

• In Scarsdale, N.Y., a prominent businessman tried to talk his college-student son out of participating in a campus demonstration. The next day, after the boy called to say he'd been arrested, the father tripped and fell down a flight of stairs. He was lucky to get off with only bruises and a badly sprained back.

• In Los Angeles, an 11-year-old girl was told that her parents were getting a divorce. At play that afternoon, she chased a ball into the street—directly into the path of an oncoming car. Fortunately, the driver braked sharply and swerved at the last moment. The girl received only cuts and contusions.

Most of us would call these incidents accidental, the results of momentary carelessness or plain bad luck. Actually, they are not. In 1938, Dr. Karl Menninger, a founder of the famed Menninger Clinic in Topeka, Kan., described such incidents as "purposive accidents"—acts which upon analysis turn out to be subconsciously motivated.

Accidents are one of the nation's major health problems. The statistics are astronomical: over 100,000 killed each year on our highways and in our homes and factories; another 360,000 permanently disabled; billions of man-hours lost; and an annual cost to industry and taxpayers in the range of $80 to $85 billion.

Obviously, it is impossible to measure exactly how much of this toll can be attributed to "purposive" accidents. They are, according to Dr. Menninger, a means that many people use to atone for guilt feelings, hostility, or frustration. Virtually every study of accidents since Dr. Menninger's early research has indicated clearly that many accidents aren't really "accidental." Moreover, if we can recognize the triggering factors, we can go a long way toward preventing future accidents.

An example is the case of Arthur Cohn, a salesclerk in a large city department store. In 1962, Cohn slipped on a newly waxed floor and sprained his ankle. Six months later, he pulled a muscle while lifting a carton. A year after that, he cut himself severely on the broken glass of a display case. Less than three months later, he was back in the first-aid office for treatment of a scalp laceration suffered when he walked into an open locker door in the employes' lounge.

On his last trip to the medical department, Cohn was interviewed by a psychiatrist. It took only two brief interview sessions to pinpoint the cause of his repeated mishaps.

An extremely passive man, Cohn is married to a particularly dominant woman. Before the most recent accident, he had had a breakfast-table argument with his wife—an argument in which he had characteristically come out on the losing end. Further analysis made him realize that all his accidents had come after similar "scenes."

This opened the door to understanding. With guidance from the doctor, Cohn began to see a pattern: unable to get back at his wife directly, he had punished himself for his weakness and, at the same time, had garnered a little sympathy by coming home with a bandage and tales of blood and pain. Once he recognized that his accidents were devices used for self-punishment and manipulation of his wife, the pattern was broken. Although his marital status hasn't changed, he has now gone several years without another mishap.

As early as 1926, a German psychologist named Karl Marbe proved statistically that a person who has had one accident is more likely to have another than an individual who hasn't had any at all. But it wasn't until the last 35 years that researchers began to probe the problem scientifically. In the late 1940s, Dr. Flanders Dunbar, a pioneer in psychosomatic medicine, interviewed patients in the accident ward of a hospital. Although all of those interviewed attributed their mishap to "uncontrollable" environmental factors, at least 80 percent revealed a significant pattern of accident-prone characteristics—all symptoms of deep emotional conflict.

A considerable amount of effort and research has been devoted to the creation of a safer environment. Such things as dual braking systems on automobiles, stronger center-strip barriers on highways, hard hats for construction workers, eye shields in factories, nonskid floor surfaces, safety-education programs, and so on, *have* served to reduce the accident rate. But current statistics show clearly that these environmental efforts are not enough.

Safety experts have been taking a long-overdue look at human factors. What they have discovered is extremely revealing.

Consider what was learned during a two-year study conducted by Dr. Harold Marcus, associate clinical professor of psychiatry at the Mt. Sinai School of Medicine in New York, at a large metropolitan department store. The survey involved one group of 26 accident-repeaters, each of whom had had at least five accidents in five years, and a second group of 26 accident-free "control" employes. All were given a battery of psychological tests, as well as at least one clinical interview.

On a superficial basis, the tests and interviews didn't turn up any marked differences between the groups. Both had their share of anxious or mildly depressed people; both revealed patterns of good and poor marital relationships. The tests and interviews turned up dramatic variations, however, in the area of basic personality, plus family background. For example:

The accident-repeater group had a predominance of passive or submissive people—and those few who could be characterized as dominant were almost all women. Among the control group, the pattern was just the opposite, with the vast majority of men dominant in their social and marital relationships.

Almost all the people in the accident group admitted to some inhibitions, guilt and fear in their attitude toward sex. In the control group, about half evaluated themselves as being completely uninhibited and free of fears in this area.

A large number of the repeaters said they were dissatsified with their jobs, while all but one of the controls said they liked their work.

There was a striking difference between the two groups in the way they handled anger. Without exception the accident-repeaters revealed that they were unable to let out anger under any circumstances; they just swallowed it. The non-accident controls, however, did a pretty good job of venting anger when it was necessary.

In the family histories of the accident group there was a formidable record of parental discord, broken homes, strict punitive discipline and poor relationships between parent and child. Although there were some broken homes in the backgrounds of the controls, most said that discipline was mild at home.

In essence, the accident-repeaters exhibited a clear pattern of suppressed anger, carelessness in work and personal habits, and passivity in all human relationships. Lacking a normal outlet for many emotions, they used self-destructive accidents as a means of expressing hostility, of getting care and attention, and as punishment for sexual guilt.

According to Dr. Harry Levinson, former director of the Division of Industrial Mental Health of the Menninger Foundation, 80 to 90 percent of all industrial mishaps can be attributed to similar psychological patterns. He points out, moreover, that the same causes probably underlie much of the sickness, absenteeism, and workplace accidents, which cost American industry some $30 billion annually.

The crucial question is obvious: Can we use these insights to *prevent* accidents? Again, consider what was demonstrated during the Marcus study. When word got around that a psychiatrist was interviewing all accident victims, the store's accident rate dropped drastically: during the study, the number of days lost because of accidents dropped 33 percent. By contrast, a program of environmental accident-prevention measures that had been instituted in the previous two years had succeeded in bringing the figure down only 14 percent.

Thus it would appear that simple recognition of accident "proneness" is a vital first step in prevention. However, beyond this there are several things a person can do to break a troublesome accident trend:

• Analyze what happened during the day that preceded an accident. Go over every event until you pinpoint the incident, or incidents, that caused anger or upset. It could be something as simple as a sharp word from the boss; or it could be guilt or hostility developing from social contacts. If you can expose the event, you may be able to recognize the reason for an accident.

• Talk out the most recent accident with a friend or relative. Plain talk can be a great release valve, and you may gain enough insight to realize that the mishap wasn't simply bad luck or clumsiness.

• Finally, there is the important role of professional help. For many people, the recognition and prevention of an accident pattern—particularly where the accidents result in serious injury—may require psychiatric assistance.

"The sum of the whole matter," Dr. Menninger has writtten, "is that our intelligence and our affections are our most dependable bulwarks against self-destruction. To recognize the existence of such a force within us is the first step toward its control."

How Quick-Witted Are You?

by Theodore Berland

ACCIDENTS don't "just happen." They happen because the situation has been set up for them, because someone has lacked an awareness of what's coming and what to do.

How do *you* react in a critical situation? Here are six emergencies that give you a chance to check your quick-wit quotient. Score yourself this way: 6 correct—you're a quick-wit; 3–5 correct—you're safe to be with; under 3—stay in bed.

The authority for Answer No. 2 is the National Marine Manufacturers Association of America; for the others it is the National Safety Council.

1. It's night. Driving along a country road, you come across a car stalled on a railroad crossing. The car is full of people, and the driver is trying to start it. You spot the light of an approaching train. What do you do?

2. You're steering your outboard motorboat, throttle open, along a deserted stream. Suddenly you spot a log in your path. Its ends almost touch both banks.

198

3. You're strolling on a sidewalk. A little girl dashes across your path and into the street after a ball—oblivious of a car speeding toward her.

4. After dusting your roses, you return to the tool shed to find your three-year-old son's hands and face covered with insecticide powder.

5. As you alight from a bus, carrying packages, the door closes behind you and you feel a tug. Your coat is caught. The bus starts to move.

6. The sky is dark, but it is a sweltering afternoon at the beach. You start swimming for a raft out in the water. When you're halfway there, rain begins to fall. You hear thunder, and flashes of lightning strike nearby.

Answers

1. Get the people out of the car immediately. Have them run a safe distance away from the tracks. Forget about the car—don't try to push it with your own; it's very difficult to estimate the speed of an oncoming train.

2. Cut the throttle! Make a sharp turn, even if it means you will beach your craft. Warn your companions to hang on, and brace yourself.

3. Yell at the child! She can stop in less distance than the car. If the child is close enough, grab her or trip her. There's one fact you should know, however: if you grab or trip the child, you assume responsibility for the consequences of the act. Nevertheless, saving a life should be uppermost.

4. Wash his hands and face with water (some pesticides can penetrate unbroken skin), grab the container (the ingredients are listed on the label) and call your poison control center or doctor. If you can't reach either, have the child drink a glass of water, and get him to a hospital right away.

5. Drop the packages, unbutton the coat and whip it off. Yell at the driver. You may have to jog a few feet if the bus starts to move, but it takes time for a bus to really get rolling.

6. Go back to shore and find shelter in a building. Don't try for the raft. Remember that lightning strikes at the highest projection; on a raft, you'd be it.

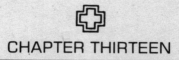

CHAPTER THIRTEEN

AN OUNCE
OF PREVENTION

Heed Your Body's Warning Signals

by Stanley L. Englebardt

A FRIEND of mine died of prostate cancer at the age of 52. Not long after, I encountered his doctor, who was our mutual friend. With a bite of anger in his voice, he told me: "Let's face it, this was probably an unnecessary death. John had months of warning symptoms, but he didn't have a check-up. An examination, performed right after he noticed changes in his urinary habits, might have saved his life."

Prostate cancer struck 73,000 Americans in 1981. One out of three of them will be dead in five years—a grim statistic. Yet the tragic fact is that many of these deaths could be prevented through early diagnosis and treatment. All told, 430,000 Americans died needlessly of various forms of cancer last year, because they didn't get treatment in time.

Why do so many people ignore the body's early-warning signs until there is no longer any hope of avoiding the full ravages of the disease? "One reason," says Dr. Thomas P. Hackett, chief of psychiatry at the Massachusetts General Hospital in Boston, who has studied hundreds of cancer cases, "is the fear of finding out that something is indeed wrong with you—something that may require hospitalization, an operation, even a change in life-style."

But fear alone isn't the only thing. Dr. Hackett found that most highly educated people—physicians and other professionals who should know that early treatment usually leads to cures—do not seek medical help any sooner than, say, a grade-school dropout. Why? "Because the person simply refuses to believe that anything unusual could be happening to him," says Dr. Hackett.

To understand why heeding early-warning signals—especially in the case of cancer—is so important, consider that cancer typically begins when a cell on the surface of tissue or in the lining of a duct undergoes an abnormal change. The rogue cell reproduces itself by dividing into two cells, which in turn redivide, on and on. Most cancers remain at the site of origin for a long time, however, before starting to invade adjacent tissues. It is during this stage that the patient has the best chance for a cure.

Although body signals are never conclusive evidence of cancer, they may be warnings that should send you to your doctor for a check-up.

Prostate cancer

This cancer usually strikes men in their middle or later years. Autopsy studies indicate that one man in five past the age of 50 has the beginnings of prostatic cancer, and cancerous changes of the prostate can be found in half of all men at age 70.

Because the prostate surrounds the neck of the bladder where it connects to the urethra, or urine-carrying tube, most symptoms are concerned with a change in urinary habits. Among these changes: the sudden need to get up during the night for urination; difficulty in starting the stream; loss of power; burning; post-urination dribbling; and sometimes dull pain in the pelvic or anal region. Although symptoms may vary, and all of them may be caused by non-malignant conditions— inflammation, infection, cysts or benign tumor—unusual urinary habits always deserve medical examination. Moreover, it's a good idea for men over 40 to have a prostate exam once a year, for prostatic cancer may spread *before* it signals.

Lung cancer

In a year, an estimated 129,000 Americans will get lung cancer, and 111,000 will die of the disease. Yet there may be loud-and-clear warning signals of an impending cancer.

To illustrate, Dr. William G. Cahan, of the Memorial Sloan-

Kettering Cancer Center in New York, pulls out the file of a 42-year-old housewife, a heavy smoker, who recently underwent surgery for removal of a lung cancer. "Her first early warning came almost three years ago when, instead of waking each morning with her usual dry, hacking 'smoker's' cough, she started raising an unusual amount of phlegm. At first she attributed this to a 'sinus condition' with a postnasal drip. She ignored it and continued smoking two-and-a-half packs of cigarettes a day.

"Most probably," says Dr. Cahan, "this transition from a dry cough signaled a change in the lining of the bronchi of her lungs. Some changes are reversible if smoking is stopped; others may progress inexorably to cancer. Too often the symptoms are misinterpreted as a chronic benign condition and allowed to progress to an inoperable state by the time medical care is sought."

The optimum time to discover lung cancer, of course, is while it is largely without symptoms. Heavy smokers should therefore have periodic chest X rays and microscopic examination of the sputum. In some instances, lung cancer can masquerade as other conditions—repeated bronchitis, frequent bouts of pneumonia, bursitis-like pain in one shoulder, angina pectoris (pain in the chest associated with heart trouble), or a significant enlargement of the area around the fingernails, called clubbing. "If the cause of any of these symptoms can't be identified," says Dr. Cahan, "the patient should have a chest X ray. This is particularly important if he or she is a heavy smoker."

Skin cancer

The most common site of cancer is the skin. Melanomas, the most deadly form of skin cancer, in some instances can be seen by the naked eye for 5 to 15 years, or even longer, before they start invading underlying tissue. During this signaling period, the condition is usually curable. Nevertheless, in 1981 5100 people died from melanoma—and 1800 more from other forms of skin cancer.

"Most melanomas start out as a seemingly normal freckle or mole," says Dr. Martin C. Mihm, a dermapathologist at the Massachusetts General Hospital and Harvard Medical School. "The patient looks at it in the mirror or bath for so long that, in effect, he stops seeing it. As a result, when the mark begins to change shape or color, it may go unnoticed."

Does this mean that all freckles and moles must be checked daily? Fortunately not. Melanoma frequently signals its onset in color changes. Go to the doctor at once if any red, white, pink or blue specks appear in a long-standing mole. Moles that are uniform bluish-black, bluish-gray or bluish-red, or of uneven surface, also deserve special medical attention. "In short," says Dr. Mihm, "simply by watching for uncharacteristic features or changes in coloring on 'moles' or 'freckles,' you can usually catch skin cancer in time."

Colon and rectal cancer

This cancer strikes 123,000 Americans a year and kills over half of them. Yet, according to the American Cancer Society, three of four could be saved by early diagnosis and treatment. Here are some signals that should be reported to your doctor at once: any change in bowel habits; any blood or mucus in the stools; any unusual crampy pains in the lower abdomen.

Uterine cancer

This cancer takes the lives of 10,000 women a year. Yet cancer in the body of the uterus frequently gives an early warning—abnormal bleeding. The best advice: let a doctor determine what the signal means—while there's a good chance, if it's cancer, for a cure. Although the cervix, or neck, of the uterus, a frequent site of cancer, may give no very early signals, cancer here can fortunately be detected in time for a complete cure in almost all cases by a "Pap" test, which should be included in every woman's regular check-up.

Breast cancer

This, too, can be headed off by self-awareness as well as regular self-examination. Among the things a woman should watch for are: any lump or thickening in the breast; alteration in the breast's contour; any discharge from the nipple. These signals can be caused by conditions other than cancer, but a doctor's definitive exam should be sought immediately.

Cancer isn't the only catastrophic disease that provides early-warning signals. Cardiologists have known for years that most heart attacks are preceded for weeks and months by a variety of subtle signs. And, if the patient is alert to these, steps can be taken to head off the event. Reviewing the experiences of hundreds of patients, Dr. Irvine H. Page, emeritus consultant cardiologist at the Cleveland Clinic, describes four primary early-warning signs: 1) The feeling that you are under constant pressure in your work and social life. 2) A buildup of classic cardiac risk factors such as overweight and high blood pressure. 3) Unaccustomed chest discomfort such as "acid indigestion," vague aching, and a feeling of fullness. 4) Overwhelming, bone-tired fatigue. "This last sign," says Dr. Page, "usually comes several hours before an actual attack. At this point you should get to a doctor immediately."

"VERY OFTEN," says Dr. Hackett, "the person in the best position to spot an early-warning sign is a mate, friend or business associate." To illustrate his point, he told me, "Two weeks ago, my wife Eleanor called and mentioned an unusual pain under her chest. She rarely talks about minor aches, so I was alerted immediately." When Mrs. Hackett added that her arms felt heavy, too, he went home at once and took her to the hospital. Examination showed that it was the start of a heart attack.

Significantly, when I asked doctors for guidance on the body's disease signals, certain words kept coming up time and again: *unusual, different, change.* "We are not suggesting that people become hypochondriacs, running to a physician for every little ache or pain," says Dr. Howard Ulfelder, Massachusetts General Hospital's deputy director of cancer services. "But any prolonged or unusual change in body patterns or functions should be checked. Chances are you'll pick up signs of disease long before it can threaten your life."

Six Ways
to Reduce
Your Cancer Risk

by Arthur C. Upton, M.D.

1. Don't smoke. This is one definite thing a person can do for himself. Two-pack-a-day cigarette smokers are at least ten times more likely to develop lung cancer than non-smokers.

2. Avoid smoke-filled places. Scientific data linking ill health to breathing "sidestream" and exhaled smoke are not as positive as smoking itself. Still, common sense suggests taking preventive action.

3. Don't get needless X rays. It is important to get X rays when they are a key part of diagnosis and treatment. But their routine use just to be sure everything checks out should be avoided.

4. Be careful of sun exposure. Risk of skin cancer can be increased by overexposure to the sun's ultraviolet light. This is especially true for people with fair complexions.

5. Avoid long exposure to household solvent cleaners, cleaning fluids, and paint thinners. Some may be hazardous if inhaled in high concentrations, particularly in unventilated areas.

6. Be careful when using pesticides, fungicides, and other garden and lawn chemicals. Follow label instructions carefully. Avoid storing or using such chemicals so that they could be inhaled or ingested, or could contaminate food, water, or toys.

What You Should Know About Eye Care

An interview with Bradley R. Straatsma, M.D.

OVER 11 million people in the United States have vision impairment. And almost one of every two Americans wears glasses or contact lenses. Here, a leading authority tells of gains in the battle to save vision— and offers helpful advice on safeguarding your own eyesight.

Q. Dr. Straatsma, are cataracts and glaucoma the main causes leading to blindness?
A. No, I'd rank those after disorders in the retina—the light-sensitive tissue at the back of the eye. One of these disorders, called macular degeneration, is a major cause of legally defined blindness. The initial symptom may be a distortion of objects. A door jamb looks crooked. Or a person may look at a word and not see one of the letters in the word. Eventually, the patient may be unable to read ordinary print.

Q. What happens then?
A. Some forms of macular disturbance disappear after a time. Other forms may be corrected by laser or surgical treatment. For still others, medical science at present does not have an effective treatment.

Q. If left untended, does macular degeneration generally result in blindness?
A. Macular degeneration can mean loss of central vision—the ability

to read and to see even the large letters on a test chart. But patients with this disorder do retain their full field of vision. Thus, they are able to move about their environment, to see left and right and up and down.

Q. Is the incidence of cataracts rising?
A. Yes, because of the age factor. About three million people in this country have some form of cataract—that is, opacity forming within the lens of the eye and gradually clouding vision. About two million of these victims are 65 or older.

Q. Has treatment of cataracts changed a great deal in the last 20 or 25 years?
A. It's one of the big steps forward in the field of ophthalmology. When surgery is necessary to remove cataract, it is safer than it was some years ago and less disruptive to patients. They can enter a hospital, have an operation the following day, and leave the hospital on the subsequent day, or in some instances undergo cataract surgery on an outpatient basis. Six to ten days of hospitalization were needed fifteen years ago.

Intraocular lens implant (replacement of the natural lens with a plastic lens) after cataract extraction is also a very important advance, and the implant is of great value for selected patients. In general, the patient is an older person, because there's greater difficulty at advancing age with contact lenses.

Q. Warnings are often heard about glaucoma. Just what is it?
A. Glaucoma is a group of diseases, all of which are characterized by an elevation of fluid pressure within the eye that destroys the delicate structures within the eye, and thus the ability to see.

Q. How does it do that?
A. The eye must maintain a certain pressure to remain healthy. With glaucoma, this normal pressure is exceeded, and the eye damaged.

Q. How is glaucoma detected?
A. The detection is aided by instruments capable of precisely mea-

suring the pressure inside the eye. If glaucoma is suspected, other tests are needed to establish the correct diagnosis.

Q. What are glaucoma's warning symptoms?

A. With the most common type of glaucoma, symptoms may be absent until the process is rather far advanced. At that point, the person may become aware of a defect in the field of vision. Rarely, there may be some cloudiness of vision. Another type of glaucoma comes on suddenly. It's associated with redness, pain, blurring of vision and the appearance of "halos" around lights.

Q. Do those symptoms tend to come and go—or would they persist?

A. In a rare form of glaucoma those symptoms may come and go. For most patients with acute glaucoma, the process begins suddenly and develops within hours into a severe disorder.

Q. Can glaucoma be treated?

A. It is generally possible with medical, and occasionally with surgical, treatment to control the process and preserve vision for the balance of the patient's life.

Q. Can you reverse damage already done?

A. No. Once part of the delicate structure of the eye has been destroyed by glaucoma, it cannot be restored.

Q. How early in life can glaucoma strike?

A. It may be present at the moment of birth, but the majority of patients develop glaucoma in adult life.

Q. How often should a person have his eyes examined, particularly for glaucoma?

A. That depends on the health of the eye, the health of the person, and the period of life. Generally speaking, I believe adults should have vision checks, with a careful medical eye examination, every two years as a reasonable minimum.

Q. What other types of eye ailments are major concerns of the medical profession?

A. One I would mention especially involves the cornea, the transparent front surface of the eye. Being exposed to the environment, the cornea is susceptible to infection—by bacteria, viruses and fungi—and to the risk of injury.

Q. How serious is the damage when this happens?

A. Initially the patient notices pain. But corneal disorders also prevent transmission of a clear image to the retina. This can cause a decrease of vision.

We are now able to treat many forms of infections effectively. Yet scars and "opacities" form. For that reason, many patients undergo corneal transplants, which have one of the best success rates of any transplantation surgery.

Q. What about other problems of the eye?

A. Oculomotor disorders affect the ability of the eye to turn in different directions and the ability of the two eyes to remain properly lined up and in focus on a particular object. This accounts for an inward turning of one eye, known as cross-eyes, or an outward turning of one eye, known as wall-eyes.

Q. Can either be corrected?

A. Yes, but a complete medical eye examination is needed because misalignment may be secondary to another ailment. Treatment may involve patching of one eye, glasses, medication, orthoptics (eye exercises and other forms of visual training) and surgery on the muscles that control the movement of the eye.

One aspect of cross-eye and wall-eye is worth emphasizing: A child, when one eye is misaligned, will suppress the image from that eye in order to avoid the symptom of double vision. In effect, he or she will be using one eye. If that process continues, particularly if it develops early in life, it becomes more and more ingrained in the child's sensory processes. When not detected and treated by a certain point in life, it may result in a permanent decrease of vision.

Thus, it's particularly important for all children to obtain an evaluation of visual acuity in the first years of life.

Q. Could a child go through the first four or five years of life with vision that tests out as normal, and then in the seventh, eighth or ninth year develop a need for glasses?
A. Yes. Just as the body changes throughout life, the eye may change in its ability to see objects sharply.

Q. How soon do children need an eye examination?
A. If there is no reason to suspect an eye problem, I recommend that examinations start at about three or four years of age. Children are then old enough to cooperate with the physician, yet young enough for many types of eye weakness to be discovered and corrected.

Q. Does watching television or reading hurt the eyes of youngsters?
A. I don't know of any indication that reasonable use of the eyes—whether for television, reading or movies—is detrimental.

Q. Are accidents a major source of eye disorders?
A. Statistically they're not as numerous as other categories, but often involve young people just when they are becoming productive. One form of accident occurring with increasing frequency is the automobile-battery explosion. Most people don't realize that the conventional car battery releases flammable materials. When a car doesn't start at night, they think nothing of lifting the hood and lighting a match. The result may be an explosion that damages one or both eyes.

Q. Can a person on the way to becoming blind or nearly blind be helped to lead a reasonably full life?
A. Yes. If the best medical science can't control the disorder, then the patient should be honestly and fully informed of his condition and given every possible assistance in making the adjustment to functioning without vision. Many people function extraordinarily well without vision.

Q. Aren't there experiments taking place in which electrodes implanted in the brain can allow a functionally blind person actually to see lines and dots?

A. There are a number of exciting developments ranging from optical devices that use magnification to devices that permit an individual without sight to "read" by means of sensations felt on a fingertip. And, yes, interesting work is being done with implanted electrodes. But we have a great deal to learn before we will be able to place this into a practical set of circumstances. Over some years, with major expenditure of time, effort, and research, we may develop a vision-substitution system for human beings.

Danger, Danger, Everywhere

by Richard Wilson

THE WORLD seems a hazardous place. Every day the newspapers announce that some chemical has been found to be carcinogenic, or some catastrophic accident has occurred. This leads some of us to hanker after a simpler world where there are fewer risks. But does such a world exist?

If we look back a century, we find that expectation of life was 50 years; now it is over 70 years. Therefore the sum of all the risks to which we are now exposed must be less than it was. Indeed, many of the large risks of the last century have been eliminated, leaving us conscious of a myriad of small ones, most of which have always existed.

The moment I climb out of bed I start taking risks. As I turn on a light I feel a tiny tingle, and I remember that every year about 1000 people are electrocuted in the United States. While taking a shower, I wonder about the chemicals the soap contains.

I ponder this risk as I walk to breakfast, taking care not to fall down the stairs. Falls kill over 13,000 people per year. Shall I drink coffee? It contains caffeine, which may be carcinogenic. Do I use sugar, which makes me fat and gives me heart disease? Or saccharin, which has caused cancer in laboratory animals?

I make a sandwich for lunch. My son likes peanut butter. Improperly stored, peanuts can develop a mold that produces aflatoxin, a potent carcinogen. I prefer meat. But a meat-heavy diet may contribute to cancer of the colon.

I live seven miles from work and can commute by car, bicycle or bus. Which has the lowest risk? Bicycle riding helps keep my weight down, and does not cause pollution—but statistics show that it is more likely to involve me in a serious accident. A car would be safer, a bus safest. I am happy that I don't have to choose between a horse and a canoe; both are even more dangerous (per mile) than a bicycle.

As I approach Boston, I see the urban haze caused by air pollution. A government laboratory reports that each year between 7500 and 120,000 people in the U.S. die because of air pollution.

I go to a committee meeting. Although I don't smoke tobacco, half of the committee members do, and I am thus exposed to the poison that annually causes 20 percent of all cancers.

At mid-morning I take a drink of water. The city's sanitation engineers use chlorine to kill bacteria in the water. By such methods the country has nearly wiped out cholera and typhus. But chlorine can react with certain organic matter in water to produce many known carcinogens. One of them, chloroform, if produced in a concentration of 100 parts per billion, presents a health hazard.

My office walls are made of cinder block, which contains radioactive materials, and radiation can increase my risk of cancer. One of these radioactive materials, radon, is a gas released by the cinder. Because I can breathe it, the hazard is accentuated. I could paint the walls with a thick coating to seal in the radon. But some paint combinations contain radioactive materials that can themselves be carcinogenic. Which is worse?

I frequently travel to distant meetings. Should I go by car, bus, train or airplane? For journeys of 1000 miles or more, train or air travel is the safest. But airplanes often fly at 30,000 feet, and at that altitude cosmic-radiation exposure is more than 60 times what it is at sea level. Even a vacation trip to the high altitudes of Colorado can increase cosmic-ray exposure. Sunlight at these altitudes, or excessive exposure even at sea level, shower us with ultraviolet light, which can cause skin cancer.

And so it goes.

THERE ARE THOSE today who would try to eliminate all known risks by law. This sounds plausible, but actually it creates an incentive for ignorance, not for safety. It would be better policy to try to measure our risks quantitatively. Then we could compare them and decide which to accept and which to reject.

To compare risks we must first calculate them. In the table below I have listed several actions that increase the chance of death in any year by roughly one in a million. How are these figured?

Take cigarettes as an example. In the United States, 627 billion cigarettes were made in 1978—enough for 3000 per person (including children). It is estimated that over 15 percent of the nearly two million Americans who die each year die prematurely from diseases caused by smoking. This is an average lifetime risk of 0.15. Dividing by the 70-year average lifetime gives a yearly risk of 0.002 or 2×10^{-3}; dividing again by 3000 gives a risk per cigarette of 0.7×10^{-6}—or, put differently, seven tenths of the one-in-a-million risk.

How can such calculations be used to eliminate risks? Well, economists are fond of using taxation to control human affairs. Why not tax anyone who introduces a risk into society? This tax could pay for medical care and compensate society for the loss of services. How much should the tax be? I suggest, as a basis for discussion, that it be at the rate of $1 million for every life that is lost by the risk in question, or one dollar for a risk of one in a million.

For example, since each cigarette increases the risk of death by 0.7 × one in a million, cigarette manufacturers would pay an increased tax of 70 cents *per cigarette*. This would be more than enough to pay the societal cost of cigarette smoking (hospital costs, fire hazards, reduced working time), which is estimated at over $1 per pack. Such taxes might be used to pay for risk reductions in other areas: for example, bringing substandard sanitation systems up to par.

Whether we quantify these risks or not, we constantly make decisions about them. We do this as individuals on a small scale; politicians do it for us on a larger scale. What we have not done, and need to do, is to compare the risks of various activities and then reduce the largest risks.

AFTER CALCULATING risks all day, I go home. Yet I still face decisions about risks. If I cook a meal in the microwave oven and the door doesn't fit tightly, I will be exposed to microwaves. It has been claimed that microwaves, even at low intensity, give people behavioral problems. Or I can use the gas stove—but if its combustion is incomplete the burning gas can fill my kitchen with both noxious carbon monoxide and nitrogen oxides.

These Actions Increase Risk of Death (per year) by One in a Million

ACTION	NATURE OF RISK
Smoking 1.4 cigarettes	Cancer, heart disease
Drinking ½ liter of wine	Cirrhosis of the liver
Spending 1 hour in a coal mine	Black lung disease
Spending 3 hours in a coal mine	Accident
Living 2 days in New York or Boston	Heart disease
Traveling 6 minutes by canoe	Accident
Traveling 10 miles by bicycle	Accident
Traveling 300 miles by car	Accident
Flying 1000 miles by jet	Accident
Flying 6000 miles by jet	Cancer caused by cosmic radiation
Living 2 months in Denver	Cancer caused by cosmic radiation
Living 2 months in a stone building	Cancer caused by natural radioactivity
One chest X ray	Cancer caused by radiation
Eating 40 tablespoons of improperly stored peanut butter	Liver cancer caused by aflatoxin
Drinking heavily chlorinated water for 1 year	Cancer caused by chloroform

I take a glass of beer. Excessive alcohol consumption may cause cirrhosis of the liver and has been associated with oral and other cancers. However, the relaxing effect of the beer reduces my stresses and permits me to have a good night's sleep. This will prolong my life and is worth the risk.

I put on my pajamas. Are they flammable? There is always a risk of a fire starting while I am in bed. As I fall asleep, I remember the truism that "more people die in bed than anywhere else." So at least I'm in the right place.

A Do-It-Yourself
Health Check-up

by Stanley L. Englebardt

AFTER First Lady Betty Ford underwent a breast-cancer operation in September 1974—followed less than three weeks later by Margaretta "Happy" Rockefeller—physicians all over the country were inundated with requests for physical check-ups. "I congratulate these people for wanting a medical examination right away," said Dr. Daniel G. Miller, medical director of the Preventive Medicine Institute-Strang Clinic in New York City. "Early detection and prompt treatment of breast cancer—and many other diseases—can mean cure or control in anywhere from 50 to 100 percent of the cases."

But early detection means just that—getting a health check-up before full-fledged disease takes over. Most of the people seeking an examination after the Ford-Rockefeller news hadn't had a complete physical in years; and many had to wait several months more before they could actually see a doctor. In fact, it has been estimated that if everyone in the United States decided to get an annual exam, instead of the one third who presently do, it would take three years for every practicing physician, working day and night, just to complete the first round. Furthermore, recent emphasis has been on self-care for disease prevention—what you can do yourself to monitor suspicious symptoms and modify risk factors.

Does this mean that we have to abandon the idea of preventive medicine through regular check-ups? "It does not," says Dr. Miller. "But it does mean that we must concentrate our resources on those who are most at risk, and testing should be done selectively, according to an individual's risk patterns for disease."

How can a person know if he's at special risk for certain diseases? The Strang Clinic has devised a self-administered health quiz. This questionnaire, it must be stressed, is not designed to *replace* a doctor's examination. "If you are currently involved in a preventive-medicine program," says Dr. Miller, "you are already following the best health course possible." But for those who haven't been getting a regular check-up, the following condensed version of the Strang do-it-yourself health quiz can be a life-saver. Answer all the questions with a yes or no. Then see the end of the article for an evaluation.

Skin and lymph nodes.

The skin is a major diagnostic aid to doctors because it mirrors, in rashes, eruptions and swollen lymph nodes, many internal diseases. Almost all skin cancer is curable if detected and treated early enough.

A. Do you now have any unexplained itching? ...... Sweating or night fever that has lasted for more than two weeks? ...... Enlargement of lymph glands? ...... Sores or growths that haven't healed in more than a month? ...... Moles that have changed color or size, have become ulcerated or bleed periodically? ......

B. Has any member of your family had cancer of the skin? ...... Lymphosarcoma or Hodgkin's disease (malignant lymph-node tumors which are often curable)? ......

C. Have you ever had a mole removed? ...... Radiation therapy? ...... A burn with scarring? ......

D. Do you sunburn easily? ......

Head and neck.

If treated soon enough, more than 80 percent of the malignancies in this part of the body have proved curable.

A. Do you now have sores or white spots in your mouth that have lasted for more than a month? ...... Hoarseness or changes in the voice? ...... Difficulty in swallowing that has lasted for more than a month? ...... Any swelling lump in the neck area? ......

B. Has a member of your family ever had cancer of the head or neck? ......

C. Have you ever had a tumor in the throat or neck? ...... A thyroid disorder? ......

D. Do you smoke cigarettes, cigars, pipe? ...... Are you a heavy drinker? ...... Do you check your mouth monthly for signs of ulcers, spots or irritations? ......

Respiratory system.

Most people are aware that lung cancer is one of the least curable of all malignancies. Yet, long before this form of cancer starts to grow, there are signals that the respiratory tract is under chronic irritation. When detected at the pre-cancerous stage, this condition is almost 100-percent curable.

A. Do you now have a cough, producing sputum, that has lasted for more than a month? ...... Sputum streaked with blood? ...... Do you get chest colds more than three times a year? ......

B. Has a member of your family ever had tuberculosis? ......

C. Have you ever had tuberculosis? ...... Chronic bronchitis? ...... Asthma? ...... Pneumonia (more than once)? ......

D. Do you smoke more than one pack of cigarettes a day? ...... Have you ever worked with radioactive materials, asbestos, coal dust or nickel, stone or other minerals? ......

Cardiovascular system.

Cardiovascular diseases are the leading cause of premature death in the United States. While it is difficult to predict with certainty those individuals who are likeliest to suffer a heart attack, there are family and living patterns which, if noted and changed early enough, can reduce one's risk.

A. Do you now have shortness of breath for no apparent reason? ...... A squeezing or pressing feeling in the mid-portion of your chest? ...... Swelling of both ankles? ...... Unexplained dizzy spells? ......

B. Has a member of your family ever had hypertension (high blood pressure)? ...... Heart attack under age 60? ...... Stroke? ......

C. Have you ever had rheumatic fever, scarlet fever, heart murmur? ...... Hypertension? ...... An abnormal blood cholesterol level? ......

D. Do you smoke cigarettes? ...... Are you obese? ...... Do you eat eggs, butter and red meat daily? ......

Urinary tract.

Recurrent infections of the urinary tract are often caused by benign or malignant growths. If detected early enough, these diseases may be cured.

A. Do you now have a more frequent urge to urinate than in years past? ...... Pain or burning on urination? ...... Blood in the urine?

B. Has any member of your family had cancer of the kidney or bladder? ......

C. Have you ever had blood in the urine? ...... Kidney stones? ...... Any chronic kidney disease? ......

D. Do you work daily with cleaning fluids, paints, dyes or benzidines? ......

Gastrointestinal tract.

Few people are able to go through life without occasional stomach upset, indigestion, diarrhea or constipation. But any such distress that persists is worthy of medical attention.

A. Do you now have heartburn, indigestion or abdominal pain that has lasted for more than a month? ...... Nausea or vomiting that has lasted for more than a week? ...... More than ten pounds of unexplained weight loss in three months or less? ...... Blood in stool (may be a tarry-black color)? ......

B. Has any member of your family had cancer of the stomach? ...... Pernicious anemia? ...... Cancer of the colon or rectum? ......

C. Have you ever had gall-bladder disorder? ...... Jaundice, hepatitis, cirrhosis of the liver? ...... Ulcerative colitis or chronic bowel problems? ......

D. Do you average more than five alcoholic drinks a day? ......

Male reproductive system.

Cancer of the prostate is such a common problem that doctors now urge every man over age 50 to have an annual prostate examination. Early diagnosis of this disease can appreciably increase the cure rate.

A. Do you now have swelling, persistent pain or discomfort in a testicle that has lasted for more than two weeks? ...... Difficulty in starting to urinate? ...... Recent problems in sexual function? ......

B. Have you ever had an undescended testicle (only one testicle in the scrotum)? ...... Inflammation of the prostate? ......

Female reproductive system.

The most successful early diagnosis test ever developed for cancer is the Pap smear, which detects cervical uterine malignancies at a time when more than 80 percent are curable. Women between 25 and 45 should have a Pap smear every two or three years; women over 45, at least once a year.

A. Do you now have bleeding between menstrual periods? ...... Bleeding after sexual intercourse? ......

B. Has any member of your mother's side of the family had cancer of the cervix, vagina, uterus or ovary? ......

C. Have you ever had an abnormal Pap smear? ...... Ovarian cyst or tumor? ...... Surgery on any female organs? ......

Breast.

Breast cancer is a leading cause of death among women today. The best protection is self-examination, followed by prompt medical examination if unusual signs are noted.

A. Do you now have breast pain not related to menstrual periods? ...... A lump in either breast? ...... Any discharge from the nipples? ...... Ulceration, puckering, scaling or any unusual change in the color or texture of the breast skin? ......

B. Has any member of your family had cancer of the breast? ...... Cysts or tumors of the breast? ......

To evaluate your answers.

In every category, the A-questions concern current symptoms. If you answer yes to any A-question, see a doctor promptly. B-questions cover family medical history; C-questions concern your own medical history; report yes answers in either B or C to your doctor at your next visit. D-questions are designed to alert you to personal health hazards; a yes here should serve as a signal to change a habit.

Beware, however, of reading extra meaning into your responses. The vast majority of yes answers will turn out to reflect nothing more than a temporary condition. Still, they can indicate an early stage of a major disease, and your prompt action *could* mean the difference between life and death.

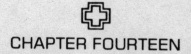

CHAPTER FOURTEEN

HOW TO COPE
WITH AN EMERGENCY

How to Recognize—and Survive— a Heart Attack

by Richard Ames

CALL this a crash program in practical cardiology. Granted, it won't tell you much about how the heart functions, or about the many kinds of heart diseases and how to treat them. But it *will* tell you how you can have a heart attack and live.

The key is knowing the Early Warning Signals (EWS) of heart attack. These are the patterns of discomfort and distress that appear in your body minutes, hours, days or even weeks before a heart attack develops. They tell you clearly, "This may be a heart attack. Get to a doctor or hospital *now*." They're worth studying. More than 550,000 Americans will die of heart attacks this year, nearly two thirds of them before they reach a hospital. At least 50,000 of these early deaths could be prevented if victims knew the EWS and received care within two hours.

Take, for example, the case of John P, who works at a service station in Springfield, Mo. Fortunately for John, the local newspapers and television stations had been carrying on an educational campaign about EWS since mid-1971. In the winter of 1972, while repairing a truck outside his garage, John felt a sensation of pressure behind his breastbone. In five minutes, the discomfort had worsened and an aching had appeared in his jaw and left arm. He went inside for a mid-morning break. But rest didn't help. In fact, by now, intense pain had also developed in his upper abdomen. He began to have difficulty breathing, and felt as if a heavy weight were pressing against the center of his chest. Suddenly, the words "heart attack" popped into his head, and with them the drawing he had seen of a man with pain spreading across his chest and running down the inside of both arms.

John grabbed the telephone and called his wife. Minutes later, they were on their way to nearby St. John's Hospital. They arrived just in time. At that moment John's heart began to fibrillate, changing from its regular rhythm into the writhing, worm-like motion that pumps no blood. When fibrillation begins, death or permanent brain damage may occur within four minutes unless normal heart rhythm is restored by electric shock, drug therapy or cardiopulmonary resuscitation. John received the first two treatments within seconds; four weeks later, he was back at work.

"What we have done with our EWS program is to take the mystery out of heart attacks," said Springfield cardiologist Glenn O. Turner, the man who spearheaded the Missouri campaign. Working with other health professionals, artists and journalists, and in cooperation with the Greene County Division of the Missouri Heart Association, Dr. Turner boiled down the very complex subject (there are, for example, more than 20 types of heart disease, and many kinds of early symptoms) into information useful to laymen.

The results have been impressive. By focusing public attention on these Early Warning Signals, the campaign has caused an increasing number of patients to call for help while there is still time. A study conducted at St. John's Hospital before and after the program began shows that during the campaign the number of patients admitted with actual or threatened heart attack increased by 20 percent, and admissions made directly into the hospital's cardiovascular-care unit increased by more than 50 percent. Before the program, the median delay between first onset of symptoms and the patient's decision to call a doctor was 4.6 hours. After the program, median delay time dropped to 2.8 hours — still, as Dr. Turner puts it, "a long way from the ideal of getting help to all patients within one hour, but nevertheless a vast improvement."

So successful has the Springfield program been that the medical community has accepted it as a national model.

Summed up Dr. Paul N. Yu, then president of the American Heart Association: "The mass education program about EWS spearheaded by Dr. Turner stands as a superb example of a practical and highly effective way to reduce the death toll from heart attacks. Know these Early Warning Signals and seek care promptly. A little knowledge is not always a dangerous thing—not when it can save your life!"

What to Do if You Feel Early Warning Signals of Heart Attack

• Call your doctor or emergency number immediately. If neither is available at once, get to the closest hospital. In calling either doctor or emergency number, emphasize that this is a heart emergency, requiring instant care; don't be put off by administrative red tape.

• When you reach the hospital, insist upon prompt care, either in the emergency room or in the coronary-care unit.

• Use the fastest transportation you can get. If you must wait even 10 or 15 minutes for an ambulance, and a car is available immediately, take the car. Don't be too concerned about bumps along the way; a moderately rough ride will not worsen your condition, but delay could be fatal. Try to get someone to drive you, and someone else to care for you on the way; but if no one is available, drive yourself, since this is less risky than remaining home alone.

• While traveling to the hospital, sit in a position most comfortable for you. Heart pain may become worse when one lies down.

• If nitroglycerin tablets are handy, place one under your tongue—it may ease pain and stress within a minute or two.

• If you are transporting the patient, watch him carefully. If he loses consciousness, and especially if his heart cannot be heard when someone holds an ear to his chest, stop the car immediately, place the patient on a hard surface outside the car, and apply cardiopulmonary resuscitation to restore blood flow and breathing. Perform these vital functions for the patient until he recovers or until an ambulance arrives. Failure to apply CPR within four minutes can cause permanent brain damage or death.

• In selecting a hospital, have two things in mind: Is it close? Is it equipped to provide truly adequate heart care? Find out now from your doctor which nearby hospital has a coronary-care unit, or at least a good emergency room, and how you can reach the hospital and be admitted without delay. The ideal is to have the patient in a good hospital within one hour of the onset of symptoms.

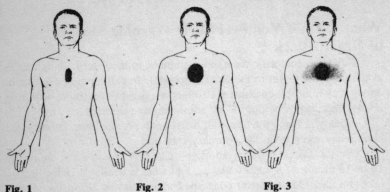

Fig. 1   Fig. 2   Fig. 3

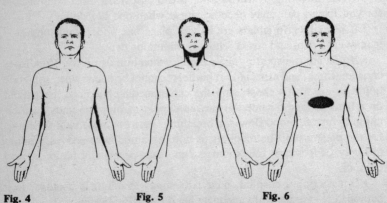

Fig. 4   Fig. 5   Fig. 6

The Early Warning Signals of Heart Attack

Figs. 1, 2, 3) The heart is in the center of the chest, not on the left, as many believe. The most common sign of heart attack is discomfort here in the center, just "under the necktie." This is usually not a sharp, jabbing pain, but a sensation of pressure, fullness, squeezing or aching. It is caused by a lack of oxygen in the heart muscle, and may be mild, moderate or severe in intensity. The discomfort may affect only the center of the chest or may radiate through the whole chest. It may subside in a few minutes or a few hours, only to return hours, days or weeks later. Don't be falsely reassured by temporary stopping of the pain; many patients have had repeated warnings of this type, but have delayed taking action until a damaging or fatal attack occurred. **Fig. 4)** Distress may extend from the chest into one or both arms or may appear in the arms alone. It may be mistaken for arthritis, bursitis or muscle strain. To tell the difference, raise your arms above your head; pain due to arthritis or bursitis will be aggravated by this maneuver, heart pain will not. **Fig. 5)** Discomfort may radiate into the neck and jaws, on one or both sides, and front or back. It may be mistaken for toothache, arthritis or "stiff neck." To test, turn your head or bend your neck; heart pain will not be aggravated, whereas most pain originating in the neck will be. Differentiation of toothache from heart attack may be more difficult; check with a doctor in case of any doubt. **Fig. 6)** Pain—usually pressure, fullness, squeezing or aching—may appear in the upper abdomen, where it is often mistaken for indigestion. Usually it is not confined strictly to the abdomen, but overlaps the lower chest at the fork of the ribs. Nausea or vomiting may occur with this pain.

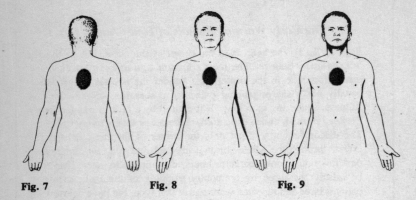

Fig. 7   **Fig. 8**   **Fig. 9**

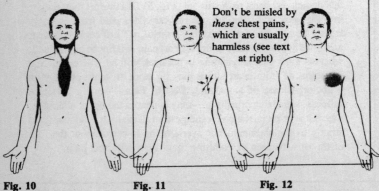

Don't be misled by *these* chest pains, which are usually harmless (see text at right)

Fig. 10   **Fig. 11**   **Fig. 12**

Fig. 7) Back pain may be the only sign of heart attack. Usually this is located between the shoulder blades, and is similar to the "tired hurt" experienced after tedious work involving protracted use of the arms and hands, and stooping of the shoulders. **Figs. 8, 9, 10)** Heart pain often occurs in a combination of patterns. The most common combinations are chest and arm pain, chest and neck and jaws, or pain in all these areas. Not infrequently, pain in the neck and jaws, abdomen, arms and back may be even more severe than that in the chest. Shortness of breath, nausea or vomiting, and heavy, cold sweating may occur with any of these combinations. Unexplained sweating, particularly if associated with pain in any of the areas just described, should always be considered a possible sign of heart attack. **Figs. 11, 12)** Pain in the left chest wall, centering on the left nipple, is almost never a sign of heart attack. This pain may be a sharp, jabbing sensation lasting a second or two, a dull soreness lasting for minutes or hours, or a combination of the two. Many tense individuals experience this pain often, and mistake it for an indication of heart disease, which it is not. It should, of course, be checked by a doctor if it persists.

CPR—
The Lifesaving Technique
Everyone Should Know

by Warren R. Young

"HELP! The man needs *help*!" The frantic cry shattered the Sunday-afternoon serenity on Seattle's Jackson Park golf course on March 26, 1972. From the elevated fifth tee, four startled high-school boys saw two youngsters hovering over the crumpled form of a man on a nearby fairway.

"Let's go!" shouted 18-year-old Craig Larson. Sprinting downhill to the stricken victim, the four boys saw that he had turned dark blue— obviously from lack of air. One of those who had shouted—15-year-old Neal Ratti, a Boy Scout—was already trying to tip the man's head back to open the air passage to his lungs. Mike Merkley, 17, quickly but carefully looked at the man's chest and dilated pupils, and felt the air in front of his nose and mouth for any signs of breath. None! Pressing fingers gently to the side of the man's Adam's apple in his neck, Mike sought any indication of a pulse. Again, none! Technically, the man was "dead."

But the boys knew that only about a minute had passed since his collapse, and that the human brain can usually survive about four to six minutes without the oxygen that the heart normally pumps to it through the bloodstream. So they set to work. Craig flopped to the ground and shoved his forearms beneath the base of the man's neck so that the others could tilt his head far enough back to assure an open air passageway past the tongue. Neal helped hold the head there while 17-

year-old Dan Fagan prepared to puff lungfuls of air into the man's mouth.

Meanwhile, Ross Venema felt the chest to locate the lower tip of the breastbone. Moving his hands an inch or two up from there, Ross placed the heel of one hand on the lower breastbone, the palm of his other hand atop the first, and began a rhythmic, strong compression of the chest, about once per second. Each time he pressed down, the man's heart was squeezed, forcing blood out to his body. With Craig calling the count, Dan inflated the victim's lungs once between every five times that Ross pressed down on his heart.

Ross was literally substituting for the victim's heartbeat; Dan was literally breathing for him. Almost magically, the man's terrible blue color began to fade away. He was alive again—although only for as long as the youths continued their successful cardiopulmonary resuscitation (CPR).

Meanwhile, another golfer had run to the clubhouse to call professional help. About eight minutes after the man's collapse, an Aid Car from a nearby firehouse slithered across the damp fairways. Two firemen took over the CPR efforts, substituting an air-bag device for the mouth-to-mouth breathing.

Ten minutes after that, an elaborately equipped hospital rescue van arrived. Using an electrocardiographic oscilloscope to monitor the victim's heart activity, electric paddles to shock his heart back into normal rhythm, plus various medications, two of Seattle's specially trained firemen-paramedics worked for 27 minutes until they achieved a slow but stable heartbeat and spontaneous breathing in the still-unconscious victim. Finally, they were able to transport him in the rescue van to the nearest hospital where a fully monitored coronary-care unit was available.

Three weeks later, the victim, a 54-year-old airline executive, walked cheerfully out of the hospital—with *no trace at all* of any permanent damage to brain or heart! A group of schoolboys, using only their own hands and exhaled breath, had brought him back from "clinical death" and safely maintained his life until more sophisticated help could come. Without their application of CPR—that combination of carefully controlled hand pressure on the chest, originated in 1960 by a Johns Hopkins University medical team, and of mouth-to-mouth breathing, developed in the late 1950s—there is no question at all but that the man's brain cells would have been irreparably destroyed.

Strangely, however, the achievement of bringing the man back to life was noted only briefly in Seattle newspapers. Why? Because that city is one of the foresighted communities across the country that have undertaken a program to make such lifesaving derring-do by ordinary citizens a matter of routine.

The model Seattle plan, jointly implemented in March 1970 by Dr. Leonard A. Cobb, chief of cardiology at Harborview Medical Center, and the then fire chief, Gordon F. Vickery, combined the city's once catch-as-catch-can rescue and emergency ambulance services into an efficient Fire Department function. A fleet of so-called Aid Cars—swift, rugged, one-ton trucks outfitted to transport patients—were readied and manned by firemen, all of whom had been trained in advanced first aid and CPR. More than 60 firemen who volunteered for 1000-hour special courses were trained as paramedical technicians at Harborview. Now these experts, in two-man teams, are poised round-the-clock to hurry to the scene of any heart attack, drowning, electrocution or sudden-death emergency in one of the five intensive-care rescue vans that have been acquired.

When a rescued patient arrives at the hospital in a van, he is moved immediately to a bed in a fully monitored coronary-care or intensive-care unit. During the first two years in which Seattle firemen ran rescue missions, about 500 sudden-death victims were treated. More than 60 of the victims were successfully revived and subsequently discharged from the hospital. "And it isn't only these clinically dead who have been saved," Dr. Cobb points out. "About 1000 other people suffering less severe forms of heart attack also got rapid assistance, thanks to the same rescue system."

Furthermore, over 200,000 Seattle adults and teen-agers have been taught to perform CPR in three-hour training courses at schools, offices, shopping centers, theaters and homes. Firemen-paramedics carefully went over the fundamentals of mouth-to-mouth respiration and external cardiac compression. Then each trainee practiced CPR on mannequins engineered to respond just like a human body.

The idea of teaching the public to bring victims of sudden death back to life by using methods which even doctors didn't know about until

1960 is clearly a dramatic, even a daring, concept. There can be pitfalls in performing CPR. For instance, if a great deal of air is blown into the stomach, it can cause trouble—even a state of near-shock. Even when done exactly right, CPR may cause cracked ribs. And when not done right, the arrow-shaped tip of the breastbone or a broken rib can puncture the liver or a lung.

The answer to these worries is proper training, in the Seattle fashion, followed by periodic refresher courses. After all, if nothing is done for a person whose heart and lungs have really stopped, death is *sure*.

Trained rescue squads and prepared coronary-care hospital units are essential prerequisites if citizen training in CPR is to reach its full potential for saving lives. Dr. Archer S. Gordon, former chairman of the American Heart Association's committee on CPR and emergency cardiac care, which developed standards for the technique, warned: "Any person who requires CPR should also have follow-up medical care." But quickness in starting CPR is equally indispensable, and even firemen cannot reach every "clinically dead" victim within minutes. If no citizen trained in CPR is at hand, a brain-damaged human being or a corpse is then the only prospect.

Hence the prestigious 20,000-member American College of Physicians recommended that a nationwide educational program be launched to teach CPR to the general public. Special emphasis would be given to training doctors, nurses, medical students, firemen, policemen, ambulance personnel and lifeguards. In addition, these specialists argued, CPR should be taught to Scouts, flight attendants, ski patrolmen, electric-utility workers, members of the armed forces, relatives of anybody with previous heart trouble—and also, in fact, to as many adults and teenagers as could be reached.

Occasions to use CPR are not likely to be rare. It is estimated that one in every six deaths in America—or about 350,000 each year—is sudden. Most of these are caused by heart attacks. Some involve drownings, electrocutions and other accidents. Autopsies of the victims in all of these categories have revealed large numbers who surely would have lived on for many years if only they had been helped past their immediate crises.

"I get a funny feeling sometimes," said one of the high-school boys who saved the Seattle golfer, "when I think how *helpless* we would have been if we hadn't been taught CPR."

Snakebite:
The Forgotten Menace

by Ben East

THE MOST dangerous animals on the North American continent are not bears, mountain lions or wolves, but poisonous snakes. Attacks occur far more frequently than most people suspect: 6500 to 7500 humans are bitten by venomous snakes in the United States each year.

Fortunately, the death rate from snakebite is low, largely because of widespread knowledge about snakes and the fact that in most cases treatment is prompt. Yet for the victims, even though they survive, the ordeal is a dreadful experience, sometimes resulting in weeks or months of illness, permanent crippling, the loss of a hand or foot, or other lasting handicaps.

Take what happened to Ray Woods on a pitch-black night in August 1957. Woods, a 50-year-old farmer living near Jamesport, Mo., was awakened around midnight by the fierce barking of his dog. Without bothering to put on shoes, he went out to the unlighted shed where the dog was tied and stepped inside to release the excited animal. As he went through the doorway, he felt something scratch or sting the instep of his right foot. He went back to the house, got a flashlight and subsequently discovered a large rattlesnake coiled just inside the shed door. He hastily applied a constricting band to his leg, and called a doctor, who arrived within 20 minutes and immediately administered antivenin snakebite serum.

In the next few hours, Woods vomited continually, or tried to, and his foot and lower leg swelled alarmingly. The swelling was accompanied by severe pain. In the next seven days, Woods' weight dropped from 210 pounds to 175. The following January, when the worst was over, he went to a Kansas City hospital for surgery to repair the injured foot. He can use it now, but large areas are still numb and he will have to wear a special shoe for the rest of his life.

Dr. Henry M. Parrish, who has devoted years to the study of snakebite, completed a countrywide survey. His findings show that the frequency of snakebite varies dramatically from state to state, depending on the prevalence of venomous snakes, the density of human population, and other factors.

Texas, home of rattlesnakes, copperheads, water moccasins and coral snakes, has more than 1400 cases annually. But when the size of human population is taken into account, North Carolina emerges as the most dangerous state in the country. In seven states, ten or more persons out of 100,000 are bitten annually. North Carolina has 19 cases per 100,000 people; Arkansas, 17; Texas, 15; Georgia, 13; West Virginia, 11; Mississippi and Louisiana, 10 each. (Despite its high rate of bites, North Carolina recorded only three deaths from 1953 through 1962, and only about 14 deaths a year occur over the entire country.) At the other end of the scale are Alaska, Hawaii and Maine, which have no native venomous snakes. The rest of New England has only a scattered population of copperheads and timber rattlers, and a correspondingly low rate of bites.

Tall tales to the contrary, the rattler, water moccasin, copperhead and coral are the only snakes north of Mexico that are dangerous to man. Of the death-dealing four, the rattlers are the most likely to be encountered. They account for something like two thirds of all snakebite cases, and the larger ones rank among the most deadly snakes on earth. Authorities list about 30 kinds, ranging in size from the 18-inch pigmy to the seven-foot diamondback. They are found in all types of habitat across the entire country, from arid desert to water holes to high timber and even near mountain snowbanks at elevations up to 11,000 feet.

The water moccasin or cottonmouth is what its name indicates—a water snake, found from Virginia to Florida to Texas, and north in a broad belt up the Mississippi Valley as far as southern Illinois. Muddy-brown or blackish, thick-bodied, and reaching a length of five feet, it is big enough to inflict a severe bite and ranks second only to the diamondback as a dangerous character. To complicate things, it resembles the harmless water snakes found in the same places, so the only safe rule in cottonmouth country is to keep away from any snake you encounter in or near water.

The copperhead is another bad actor of wide range, scattered from New England to Kansas and Georgia to Texas. In the North, it prefers rocky, timbered hillsides and stone walls, but in the South it can be happy in a swamp. It grows to a length of three feet and can also deliver a fatal bite.

The rattler, water moccasin and copperhead are pit vipers, easy to identify—provided you get close enough—by a deep pit on each side of the head between eye and nostril. The coral snake, a relative of the cobra and other killer snakes of Asia, Africa and Australia, is readily recognized by its bright-red, black and yellow coloring. It is found only in the South, from North Carolina to the Gulf and west to Texas. Small (20 to 30 inches) and a burrower, it spends much time underground or beneath dead logs, and accounts for fewer than one in 100 cases of snakebite. The fangs of a full-grown coral snake are less than a quarter of an inch long, while a big rattlesnake's are close to a full inch. As a result, the coral's bite is shallow, and delivers a very small dose of venom. But the venom is many times as toxic as that of the pit vipers. Whereas 140 milligrams of venom from a western diamondback constitute a lethal dose for a man, only five milligrams of coral-snake venom can be fatal, paralyzing the diaphragm.

Many precautions, such as snakeproof boots, will lessen the risk of being bitten. But the surest way to miss snakebite is to stay alert to the danger. Remember that a venomous snake usually hunts at night and can strike one third of its own length, lashing out at you like a steel spring unhooked. Don't depend on rattlers to rattle before they strike: some do, some don't. Don't pick up or handle any snake, dead or alive, until you are positive it is not venomous. "Dead" reptiles have a way of coming to life, and the severed head of a freshly killed snake is fully capable of delivering a bad bite. Even very young snakes have effective poison equipment—though, other factors being equal, the bigger snake is more dangerous, injecting more venom and driving it deeper.

More persons are bitten in their own yards than in any other place. Buildings with broken walls and a crawl space under the floor are especially likely to attract rattlers and copperheads. A snake hunter in South Dakota once took eight prairie rattlers from beneath a farmhouse occupied by an elderly woman. Mice were the attraction in that case, as they often are. Farm workers are frequently struck, as are people picking up logs or rocks. Woodpiles, rubbish heaps and hen houses are danger spots. And fishermen are victims more frequently than hunters, for the obvious reason that most snakes are inactive from fall to spring.

Since first-aid treatment for snakebite is painful and can cause infection, the first thing to do is determine, positively, whether it's needed. Here is what you should do:

1. The most important thing is to get the victim to a hospital immediately. Remain calm. Keep the victim as still as possible to slow the spread of venom. If you are alone and in remote country, walk—don't run—for help. If the hospital can be reached in four to five hours and no symptoms occur, no further first-aid measures are necessary.

2. If the victim shows moderate symptoms (mild swelling, pain or discoloration at the site of the wound, tingling sensations, rapid pulse, weakness, dimness of vision, nausea, vomiting or shortness of breath), tie a lightly constricting band at least three quarters to 1½ inches wide, 2 to 4 inches above the bite. *Never* use a band around a joint, the head, neck or trunk. Don't make it so tight that you can't get a finger under it.

3. If the victim shows severe symptoms (rapid swelling, intense pain at the site of the wound, blurred vision, possibly paralysis or convulsions) and you can't get medical help at once, perform cut and suck. Make a lengthwise incision ¼ to ½ inch long through each fang mark and slightly beyond it. Make the cut very shallow and cut only the skin. *Never* make a cut on the head, neck or trunk. If you have a snakebite kit, apply a suction cup over the wound. Otherwise, you should suck out as much blood and venom as you can by mouth. There is no danger from any small amount of venom that might be swallowed since it is quickly neutralized in the stomach. However, it is best to spit it out and, if possible, rinse the mouth with water.

4. Remember: *Never apply cold therapy* and don't give the victim any alcohol or medication.

Of course, the best thing to do about snakebite is to avoid being bitten in the first place. But if you fail in this, prompt and proper treatment will make the suffering less terrible—and can spell the difference between living and dying.

The Heimlich Maneuver: Help for the Choking Victim

by Andrew Hamilton

AT LEAST EIGHT AMERICANS choke to death every day on food and other objects stuck in their throats. Choking can be confused with heart attack (the choking victim cannot speak or breathe; he turns blue, then becomes unconscious) and nothing is done except to call a doctor. From the moment that an object is lodged in the windpipe and cuts off oxygen, the victim has four or five minutes to live.

Now, an easy-to-apply technique—the Heimlich Maneuver—can help. Developed in 1974 by Dr. Henry J. Heimlich, director of surgery at Jewish Hospital in Cincinnati, the technique involves sudden compression of the lungs to increase air pressure within the trachea and eject the object in the throat.

The following procedures are recommended by Dr. Heimlich and have been endorsed by the American Medical Association:

If the victim is standing or sitting: Position yourself behind him, wrap your arms around his waist. Make a fist with one of your hands and place it, thumb-side in, slightly above the victim's navel and below the rib cage. Grasp the fist with your other hand and press into his abdomen with a quick upward thrust. Repeat several times, if necessary, until the object is ejected.

If the victim is lying down: Place him face up and kneel astride his hips. With one of your hands on top of the other, place the heel of the

245

bottom hand on the abdomen slightly above the navel and below the rib cage. Press into the abdomen with a quick upward thrust.

If you are alone and choking: Try anything that applies force just below your diaphragm. Press into a table or a sink, or use your own fist.

The Heimlich Maneuver may crack a rib or cause slight internal damage, but the danger is a minor problem when a life is saved.

Reader's Digest®

Handbook of FIRST AID

Edited by
Lois Mattox Miller and
Susan W. Thompson
Reader's Digest Staff Consultants

Medical Consultants

DR. LEONA BAUMGARTNER
Former New York City Commissioner of Health

DR. RALSTON R. HANNAS, JR.
Director, Emergency Services, St. Joseph Hospital, Kansas City, Mo.
Past President, American College of Emergency Physicians

DR. JAMES J. DINEEN
Director, Emergency Training Programs,
Department of Continuing Education, Harvard Medical School

Prologue

WHEN SOMEONE is injured or suddenly becomes ill, there is a critical period—before you can get medical help—that is of the utmost importance to the victim. What you do, or what you don't do, in that interval can mean the difference between life and death. For serious conditions it is vitally important *to get* the patient to a doctor. You will always find one at the emergency facility of the nearest hospital. If you cannot take the patient there, call an ambulance at once.

First aid is the help that you can provide until professional help takes over. You owe it to yourself, your family and your neighbors to know and to understand procedures that you can apply quickly and intelligently, in an emergency.

The Reader's Digest Handbook of First Aid gives you that important information in concise, convenient form. Read and study the contents carefully; then place it with your first-aid kit or keep it in a convenient place where it will be at hand for quick reference when needed.

Table of Contents

Reader's Digest Handbook of First Aid

Prologue   248

First Steps in First Aid   251

First-Aid Procedures (in alphabetical order)   252

Warning on Drugs   289

First-Aid Kit   289

Checklist of Supplies   290

Index   293

Emergency Telephone Numbers   291

FIRST STEPS IN FIRST AID

1. The first thing to think of when you approach a seriously injured person is the ABCs:

A is for Airway. Make sure the victim's airway has not been blocked by the tongue, secretions or some foreign body (see page 258).

B is for Breathing. Make sure the person is breathing. If not, administer artificial respiration (see page 258).

C is for Circulation. Make sure the patient has a pulse. If no pulse is felt, administer cardiopulmonary resuscitation—CPR (see page 261).

2. Check for bleeding.

3. Act fast if the victim is bleeding severely (see page 257), or if he has swallowed poison (see page 284), or if his heart or breathing has stopped. Every second counts.

4. Although most injured persons can be safely moved, remember that it is vitally important not to move a person with serious injuries of the neck or back, unless it is necessary to save him from further danger (see pages 253 and 282).

5. Keep the patient lying down and quiet. If he has vomited—and there is no danger that his neck is broken (see page 265)—turn him on his side to prevent choking. Keep him warm with blankets or coats, but don't overheat him or apply external heat.

6. Have someone call for medical assistance while you apply first aid. The person who summons help should tell the nature of the emergency and ask what should be done pending the arrival of the ambulance.

7. Examine the victim gently. *Cut* clothing, if necessary, to avoid abrupt movement or added pain. Don't pull clothing away from burns unless it's still smoldering (see pages 265 and 266).

8. Reassure the victim, and try to remain calm yourself. Your calmness can allay his fear and panic.

9. Don't give fluids to an unconscious or semiconscious person; fluids may enter the windpipe and cause strangulation. Don't try to arouse an unconscious person by slapping or shaking.

10. Look for an emergency medical identification card, or an emblematic device that the victim may be wearing to alert you to any health problems—allergies or diseases that require special care.

Note on Cardiopulmonary Resuscitation

This lifesaving technique requires training, skill, and practice. To be prepared for emergency, at least one member of every family should seek instruction (see pages 236–239). The untrained may cause serious damage to the patient.

AUTOMOBILE ACCIDENTS

NOTHING IS LIKELY to test one's knowledge of first aid more than accidents suffered on the highway. Injuries may be severe; you may be a great distance from professional help. Keep a copy of this handbook in your car, along with adequate emergency supplies. The following supplies are recommended:

• Wooden splints (or inflatable ones) obtainable from surgical-supply stores or from lumber suppliers—several measuring ¼ × 4 × 36 inches (½ × 10 × 91 cm.) and several ¼ × 4 × 18 inches (½ × 10 × 46 cm.).

• At least three roller bandages 3 inches × 5 yards (8 cm. × 5 cm.): three squares of cloth 42 × 42 inches (107 × 107 cm.) to make triangular bandages or slings. A supply of safety pins 1½ inches (4 cm.) long to hold the triangular bandages in place.

• A box of twelve sterile dressings 4 × 4 inch (10 × 10 cm.) and two rolls of adhesive tape 1 inch and 2 inches (3 and 5 cm.) wide.

• Blankets to keep the injured person covered and to move him (see page 282).

• A good flashlight with fresh batteries, and warning lights or flares to be used if car is stalled.

In giving first aid, remember that moving the victim, making a hasty attempt to get him out of the car, may do untold harm, particularly if spinal injuries or leg fractures are involved.

Give first aid at once, *inside the vehicle whenever possible*, before attempting to move the injured person. Exceptions: (a) when the vehicle is on fire; (b) when gasoline has been spilled and fire hazard is great; (c) when you are in a congested high-speed area where there is a danger of a second accident. Follow these rules in examining the patient:

1. Assure that the victim is breathing and has a pulse (see pages 258–263).

2. Check for hemorrhage (see pages 257, 279).

3. Examine for injuries, particularly fractures.

4. Apply appropriate first-aid measures.

5. In case of fractures, wait for medical help. Or, if the patient must be moved to get help, follow the suggested procedures for dealing with fractures (see page 264) and for moving injured persons (see page 282).

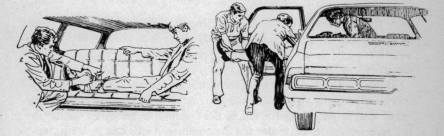

BITES—ANIMAL

WASH THE WOUND immediately with water, to flush out the animal's saliva. Then cleanse the wound for five minutes with plenty of soap and water. Rinse thoroughly and cover with a dressing or clean cloth.

Consult a doctor immediately. He will treat the wound more effectively and decide what measures are necessary to guard against rabies and tetanus infection.

If the bite is from an unknown dog, cat, or other animal, call the police to have the animal caught and observed for rabies. If the animal disappears, or if observation shows that it has rabies, the victim may need anti-rabies injections.

BITES—ANT, CHIGGER, MOSQUITO

WASH THE AFFECTED PARTS with soap and water. Apply a paste made of baking soda and a little water, or use calamine lotion. (Chiggers don't attach themselves firmly for an hour or more. Scrubbing with a brush and soapy water promptly after exposure should remove them.) If there is swelling, cover the bite with a cloth saturated with ice water. An allergic reaction to ant bite can be serious, occasionally fatal. Follow instructions for reaction to stings (see page 286).

BITES—TICK

DON'T TRY to tear an embedded tick loose. Usually you can dislodge it with a few drops of turpentine. Or cover it with a heavy oil or petroleum jelly to close its breathing pores; often this will cause it to disengage within a half-hour.

If this doesn't work, remove the tick with tweezers, working gently and slowly so that you don't crush the insect and so that all parts of its head come loose. (Avoid touching ticks with your hands.) Then scrub the area with soap and water for five minutes. Ticks can transmit dangerous disease, but usually don't if removed soon after they've become attached. If the bite becomes inflamed and swollen, or if the patient has a fever, notify a doctor.

BITES—VENOMOUS SNAKES

The best treatment for snakebite is prevention.

The dangerous venomous snakes in the United States are rattlesnakes, copperheads, water mocassins and coral snakes. More than half of the cases of venomous snakebite occur in Texas, North Carolina, Florida, Georgia, Louisiana and Arkansas.

If you live, work, or vacation in venomous-snake country, avoid infested areas. If you must enter such areas, wear protective clothing— mid-calf boots, long pants, and gloves that cover your forearms. Find out in advance of entering snake areas where the nearest medical facility is located. Read up on snakes, their habits and how to avoid their bites.

TO HELP A PERSON BITTEN BY A VENOMOUS SNAKE:

Take the victim to the nearest hospital at once. En route, keep the person as still as possible, preferably in a reclining position (to slow blood circulation and the spread of the venom). Keep the wound at or below heart level. If the hospital can be reached within four to five hours, and no symptoms occur, no other measures are necessary. *Do not apply ice or any cold therapy. Don't give medication or alcohol.*

Be alert for the development of symptoms. These will determine whether the following first-aid procedures are needed.

CONSTRICTING BAND

If the bite is on an arm or a leg and the victim experiences moderate symptoms (mild swelling, pain or discoloration at the site of the wound, tingling sensations, rapid but strong pulse, weakness, nausea and vomiting, dimness of vision, shortness of breath), apply a lightly constricting band 2 to 4 inches (5 to 10 cm.) above the bite. *Never use the band around a joint, the head, neck or trunk.*

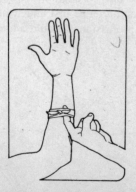

The constricting band should be at least ¾ to 1½ inches (roughly 2 to 4 cm.) wide. Tie it just tight enough to retard the spread of venom, but not so tight that it shuts off deep-lying circulation of the blood. If the band is properly adjusted, you should be able to slip your finger under it (see illustration, page 255). With the band in place, proceed with appropriate speed to the medical facility.

INCISION AND SUCTION

If the person bitten on an arm or leg suffers any severe symptoms— rapid swelling, numbness and intense pain at the wound site, rapid but weak pulse, blurred vision, convulsions, or paralysis—and you are unable to transport the victim to a hospital or get professional help at once, perform incision and suction. Follow these steps:

1. With the victim lying down, place a constricting band above the wound if you have not already done so (see directions on page 255).
2. Sterilize a knife or razor blade in a flame (several matches will do). Then, taking care to cut *only the skin*, make a lengthwise incision ¼ to ½ inch long (½ to 1¼ cm.), through each fang mark and extending slightly beyond it. (Because the snake strikes downward, its venom is usually deposited slightly beyond the puncture wound.) (See illustration below.) *Caution*: Do not make incisions on the head, neck, trunk. If the bite is on the victim's fingers or toes, take extreme care to make incision *only through the skin*. Because of the network of nerves, tendons and arteries just under the surface of the skin in these areas, only a professional should attempt incision.

BLEEDING—SEVERE

1. Have victim lie down to prevent fainting. To stop the bleeding, place a sterile gauze dressing (or the cleanest cloth item available) over the wound and *with the palm of your hand press it firmly*. If the dressing becomes saturated with blood, lay a fresh one directly over it and continue pressure. If the wound is on the head, neck, arm or leg, and there's no suspected fracture, elevate it—to a level above that of the heart—to help stop the bleeding while you apply direct pressure.

2. If bleeding from an arm or leg cannot be stopped by elevation and direct pressure over the wound, try shutting off circulation in the main blood-supplying artery by pressing it firmly with your fingers against the underlying bone. Keep your fingers straight—not curved—for this technique. There are four points where arterial pressure is practical for first-aiders (see below). But don't try arterial pressure for wounds of the head, neck or torso.

3. When the bleeding stops, bandage the dressings firmly in place—but not so tightly that you can't feel the pulse below or beyond the wound. Call the doctor, and leave the cleaning and treatment of the wound to him. Watch carefully for signs of shock (see page 285).

To prevent infection, avoid, if possible, touching any wound with an unsterilized covering or your unscrubbed hands. But in an emergency you may have no choice. The average adult has five to six quarts of blood; loss of more than two or three pints can be serious. So you may have to act fast and use whatever is available.

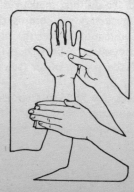

BLISTERS

THE UNBROKEN SKIN covering a blister affords the best protection against infection.

If a blister has broken, wash the area gently with soap and water, and cover with a sterile dressing.

BREATHING STOPPED—ARTIFICIAL RESPIRATION

Do the following in rapid succession:

1. Open the airway: unless you suspect a broken neck, place the victim on his back. Wipe any foreign substance—solid or liquid—out of his mouth with your fingers. If the neck is not broken, put one hand under the victim's neck and lift it up. Place your other hand on the forehead and tilt the head back so that the chin points straight up (see illustration page 259). This position prevents obstruction of the airway by the tongue. (When, in an unconscious person, the lower jaw falls backward, the tongue also falls back and obstructs the throat.)

   Opening the airway may start the person breathing again. Watch the chest for rise and fall. Listen for the sound of breathing. Place your cheek close to the victim's mouth and nose to feel any exhaled air (see illustration page 259). If there is none, take step 2 at once:

2. Pinch the nostrils closed. (Use the thumb and index finger of the hand that is on the victim's head. To do this, maneuver your hand so that it continues to exert the necessary pressure on the head to maintain the proper tilt.) Place your mouth over the victim's and blow hard four times in rapid succession, pausing between breaths only long enough to take another deep gulp of air (see illustration page 260). Then quickly take step 3:

3. Feel the carotid pulse in the neck for at least five seconds (see illustration on page 260) and instructions in the box. If there is a pulse but still no breathing, begin step 4—steady mouth-to-mouth breathing:

4. With the victim's head tilted as in step 1, and the nose pinched shut, place your mouth over the victim's and blow hard. Remove your mouth to allow the victim to exhale and you to take another deep breath. Watch for the rise and fall of the chest and listen for the sound of exhaled air. Then blow again. Repeat this procedure, giving one vigorous breath every five seconds until the victim starts to breathe spontaneously or until help arrives. Do not give up. Have someone call an ambulance or emergency rescue squad as soon as you can. Place a blanket or coat over the person for warmth *if necessary*. When the person revives, don't let him get up. Keep him lying down during transportation to the hospital emergency facility.

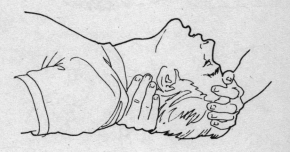

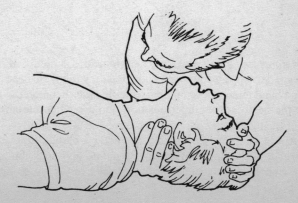

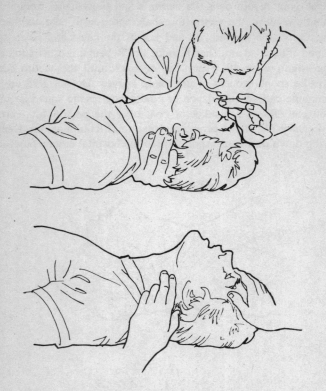

For infants and small children, the procedure is modified. To open the airway, don't place your hand under the neck to tilt the head. Instead, place one hand under the shoulders. Put the other hand on the forehead to keep the head in the proper position. Do not pinch the nose closed but cover the mouth *and nose* with your mouth. Blow gently—use only light puffs of air, not full breaths, to inflate a child's lungs. Feel the pulse over the left nipple. If there is a pulse, give one gentle puff of air once every three seconds for an infant; every four seconds for a child.

If you suspect the victim's neck is broken—a definite possibility in drowning and water accidents, or in those involving large scalp wounds or facial injuries—avoid all movement of the neck. To open the airway, place a hand on each side of the victim's head to maintain it in a neutral position. Then use the index fingers to move the lower jaw forward, without moving the head or neck. (It may be easier to use mouth-to-nose respiration. Place your cheek over the victim's mouth and breathe into his nose.)

Caution: Some 25,000 Americans have had their larynxes surgically removed and can breathe only through an opening in the neck called a stoma. In such cases artificial respiration must be performed mouth-to-stoma.

It is not difficult to locate the pulse in the carotid artery. It can be felt on either side of the neck. Locate the Adam's apple (the larynx), then slide the tips of your index and middle fingers gently into the groove between the Adam's apple and the muscles of the neck. Practice locating your own pulse so you'll be ready in an emergency. Don't compress the pulse area—touch it softly.

BREATHING STOPPED, NO PULSE—CARDIOPULMONARY RESUSCITATION (CPR)

REMEMBER THE ABCs (SEE PAGE 251). Make certain that the airway is clear; give four quick breaths, and feel the carotid pulse (see above).

If there is no pulse, the heart has stopped. While someone summons an ambulance, cardiopulmonary resuscitation (CPR) must be started at once. CPR is the combination of artificial respiration and artificial circulation—external heart compression.

With the victim stretched flat on his back on the ground or floor, kneel beside him and position his head to keep the chin up and the airway open (see illustration below).

Feel the chest to locate the lower tip of the victim's breastbone. Place two fingers of your left hand on the tip. Move the heel of the right hand (never the palm) against the fingers. (The heel will be about 1½ inches (4 cm.) above the tip and over the lower third of the breastbone. Then place the left hand atop the right. (If you're left-handed, reverse the hand instructions.)

Position your body so that your shoulders are directly above your hands, with your arms straight and elbows locked (see illustration below).

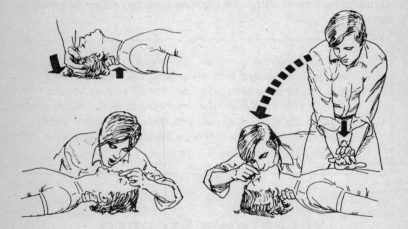

With a smooth, firm thrust, push down. Use sufficient force to press the lower one-third of the breastbone down at least 1½ to 2 inches (4 to 5 cm.), letting your back and body do the work. Then lift your weight, relaxing pressure completely. Do not remove your hands from the victim's chest when you relax between compressions. Never press the tip of the breastbone. Do not allow your fingers to press on the chest. If you interlock your fingers, this is easier.

If you are alone, repeat this rhythmic compression: press...release...press...release...80 times a minute. Each time you bear down, you squeeze the victim's heart, forcing blood out to his body, literally substituting for his heartbeat. If you are alone with the victim, stop after each 15 compressions and give two quick breaths. Continue this 15-to-2 rhythm until the pulse returns or help comes.

If someone can assist you, have the aide kneel at the victim's head and give mouth-to-mouth respiration at the rate of one breath for each five compressions you perform. This means that you, not forced to stop compressions to interpose breaths, perform compressions at the rate of 60 per minute.

To help maintain proper timing, count in this style if you are alone: "one-and, two-and, three-and . . ." until you have done the required compressions. For two-person CPR, count: one, one thousand; two, one thousand; three, one thousand; four, one thousand; five, *breathe*. Remember the rule: For one rescuer—the ratio of compressions to breaths is 15:2. For two rescuers—5:1.

CPR FOR INFANTS AND SMALL CHILDREN.

Clear airway. See special instructions (page 260). Feel pulse over the left nipple. For compression of the infant's heart use only the tips of the index and middle fingers on *one* hand. For infants under one year old, the compression rate is 100 times per minute. Press the middle of the breastbone, depressing it only ½ to 1 inch (about 1¼ to 2½ cm.). Give one small breath after each five compressions.

For small children—one to eight years old—the compression rate is 80 per minute. Use the heel of one hand or as many fingers as are necessary to press down the breastbone. Depress the breastbone 1 to 1½ inches (2½ to 4 cm.). Administer one small breath after each five compressions.

Caution: Medical groups advise against the performance of CPR by untrained persons. Even when expertly done, CPR may cause cracked ribs. When incorrectly done, the tip of the breastbone or a broken rib can puncture the liver or a lung. Hence, proper training in the technique is urged.

Instruction may be obtained at the local Red Cross, Heart Association, or other local agencies. Ask your hospital where to go in your community. *Without CPR* anyone whose heart has stopped will die, so in an emergency it may be necessary to perform CPR even if you have not been trained or certified.

BROKEN BONES

KEEP THE BROKEN BONE ends and adjacent joints from moving. Maintain the victim's body temperature and, if necessary, treat for shock (see page 285). If a broken bone protrudes through the skin and there is severe bleeding, stop the bleeding (see page 257), but do not attempt to push the bone back in place. Make no attempt to clean the wound. Summon emergency medical assistance at once.

Don't attempt to move the patient if the break is in the back, neck, pelvis, or skull. (See "Broken Neck or Back," next, and "Head Injury," page 279.) If the victim of a less serious fracture must be moved to receive medical aid, immobilize the fracture with splints to prevent further damage. (Don't assume that no bones are broken merely because the victim can move the injured limb or joint.)

For splints, use anything that will keep the broken bones from moving—newspapers, magazines, broomsticks or boards for arms or legs. Make the splints long enough to reach beyond the joint above and below the break. Apply an insulated ice bag to the injured area to relieve pain.

In auto accidents, splint a fractured leg, if possible, before moving the victim from the car. Place cloth padding between the legs. Then, using bandages or other material, tie the injured leg to the uninjured leg above and below the fractured site, and immobilize it as much as possible with an improvised short splint.

Arm or leg splinting is done merely to immobilize the break. Leave bone-setting to the doctor and splint the limb in the position in which you found it. If it is impossible to apply a splint without straightening

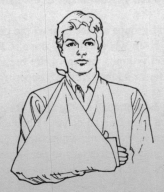

the limb, support it with a hand on either side of the break while someone gently eases it into a position as nearly natural as possible. Pad improvised splints with cotton or clean rags and tie them snugly (but not too tightly) in place with bandages, belts, neckties or strips of clothing.

BROKEN NECK OR BACK

IF THE VICTIM cannot move his fingers readily, or if there is tingling or numbness around his shoulders, his neck may be broken.

If he can move his fingers but not his feet or toes, or if he has tingling or numbness in his legs, or pain when he tries to move his back or neck, his back may be broken. Summon emergency medical assistance at once.

Don't move the victim or let him try to move. The spinal cord extends down through the neck and back vertebrae, and any movement may cause paralysis.

If the victim is not breathing, administer artificial respiration, taking care to avoid *all movement of the neck* (see page 258). *If, to avoid further injury, the victim must be moved*, carefully support his head and neck and *move him lengthwise—not sidewise* (see illustration, page 282).

Maintain normal body temperature. Carefully loosen restrictive clothing around the victim's neck and waist.

BRUISES—INCLUDING BLACK EYE

PLACE AN INSULATED ICE BAG or cold compress (a small towel soaked in ice water and wrung out) over the bruise. This should reduce both the pain and the swelling. If the pain persists, or if vision is impaired, take the patient to a doctor.

BURNS—CHEMICAL

FLUSH THE BURNED AREA copiously with running water to dilute and remove the chemical. Then treat as you would a comparable burn from any other cause (see page 266).

If an eye is burned by a chemical, especially by an acid or a basic substance like lye, flush it at once gently but thoroughly with running water for 15 minutes. Cover both eyes with gauze or a clean cloth. (Otherwise, when the uninjured eye moves, the injured eye will also.) Have the eye checked at once by a doctor.

BURNS AND SCALDS—MAJOR

1. If the victim's clothing is on fire, or still smoldering, stop the burning by rolling him on the ground. Douse him with water or smother the flames with coat, blanket or rug.
2. Keep the victim lying down, to lessen shock.
3. Cut clothing away from the burned area. If cloth adheres to the burn, don't pull it loose; leave it and cut gently around it.
4. Call for medical assistance immediately or move the victim to the nearest hospital facility.
5. Cover the burn with a sterile dressing or clean sheet. This excludes air, reduces pain and risk of contamination. Don't apply burn ointments, oil or antiseptic of any sort, and don't attempt to change the dressings.

BURNS AND SCALDS—MINOR

SUBMERGE THE BURNED SKIN immediately in cold water. On burns that cannot be immersed, apply cloths soaked in ice water, and change them constantly. Continue treatment until pain is gone. Avoid ointments, greases and baking soda, especially on burns severe enough to require medical treatment. Doctors must always scrape off such applications, which delays treatment and can be extremely painful. If the skin is blistered, cover the burn with sterile dressings. Don't break or drain blisters.

Caution: Even superficial burns or scalds may be dangerous if large areas are involved. A burn on the face, hands, feet or genitalia should be considered a major burn. Consult a physician.

CARBON-MONOXIDE POISONING

CARBON MONOXIDE is a colorless, odorless gas that kills without warning. A car engine left running in a closed garage can swiftly produce a lethal dose of carbon monoxide. The gas is also generated by wood, coal and charcoal fires, faulty oil burners, etc. In poorly ventilated rooms, the hazard of poisoning is present.

Symptoms of carbon-monoxide poisoning are: headache, dizziness, weakness, difficult breathing, possible vomiting, followed by collapse and unconsciousness. Skin, fingernails and lips may be pink or cherry-red.

First aid: Open all windows and doors and get the victim into open air immediately. Begin artificial respiration promptly (see page 258) if he is not breathing or is breathing irregularly, and cardiopulmonary resuscitation (see page 261) if his heart has stopped. Keep him lying quietly to prevent shock. Maintain normal body temperature. Call the doctor, hospital, fire department or police emergency squad. Be sure to state the nature of the trouble and specify the need for oxygen because of carbon-monoxide poisoning.

CHILDBIRTH—EMERGENCY

CHILDBIRTH is natural and normal. Let nature take its course. Do not hurry the birth; do not interfere with it. Wash your hands; keep the surroundings as clean as possible. During the birth process, only support the emerging baby. Keep hands and tools out of the birth canal.

- When the head emerges, observe the baby's neck. If, as sometimes happens, the umbilical cord is wrapped around the neck, gently slip it over the baby's head. *Do not hurry to cut the cord.*

- When the baby has been delivered, check breathing. Clean debris from mouth with a bit of gauze (or a finger-sweep will do) and, if necessary, give mouth-to-nose respiration (see page 260). Be gentle.

- Place the baby between the mother's thighs (with baby's head slightly lower than his trunk), or at the mother's side at a level no higher than her heart, until the umbilical cord is cut. Cover the baby for warmth.

- Gently massage the mother's abdomen to help her uterus contract.

- Do not wash white material off the baby; it protects the skin.

- Do nothing to baby's eyes, ears and nose.

- *Cutting the Umbilical Cord.* If the mother can be taken promptly to the hospital, no harm will result if the infant remains attached to the afterbirth by the umbilical cord until the mother arrives at the hospital. But if you must cut the cord, wait until it is limp and pulseless, or the afterbirth has been expelled.

Tie a clean tape or cloth in a square knot around the umbilical cord about four inches (10 cm.) from the baby. Tie a second tape around the cord about four inches (10 cm.) from the first knot. If no tapes are available, shoestrings may be used. Immerse scissors in boiling water, or clean them in alcohol. Then cut the cord between the two tapes.

- Notify the mother's physician and transport mother and child to the appropriate hospital.

This article is adapted from the American Medical Association's First-Aid Guide.

CHOKING, WHILE EATING

THE HEIMLICH MANEUVER (also called the abdominal thrust) is the most effective of the first-aid measures for choking. Choking means that something—food or a foreign body—is plugging the victim's windpipe so that he cannot breathe. If the airway is completely blocked, the victim, unless relieved of the obstruction, may die in less than five minutes. You must act fast.

First, make sure the person is choking and not having a heart attack. If a person who is eating suddenly looks startled, puts his hand to throat, cannot speak or breathe or begins to turn blue, *quickly* ask him if he is choking. If he is unable to speak and nods his head "yes," apply the Heimlich Maneuver.

TO APPLY THE HEIMLICH MANEUVER

If the victim is standing or sitting, stand behind him and extend both arms around his waist (see illustration below).

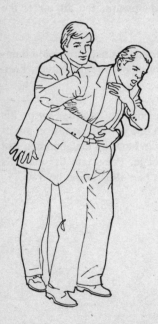

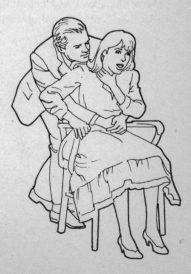

- Make a fist with one hand and place the thumb-side against the victim's abdomen, slightly above the navel and below the rib cage.

- Grasp your fist with the other hand and press it forcefully into the abdomen with a quick upward thrust. Repeat several times if necessary.

(The maneuver works on the principle that there is always some residual air trapped in the lungs of the victim. When compressed by pressure below the diaphragm and forced upward, the air ejects the obstruction caught in the windpipe.)

Caution: Don't squeeze the person with your arms. This could damage the ribs. To avoid squeezing when you apply the maneuver, keep your arms bent at the elbows.

- If the choking victim is lying down, position him *face up* on his back and kneel astride his hips. With one of your hands on top of the other, place the *heel* of your bottom hand on the abdomen just above the navel and below the rib cage. Press into the victim's abdomen with a quick upward thrust (see illustration below).

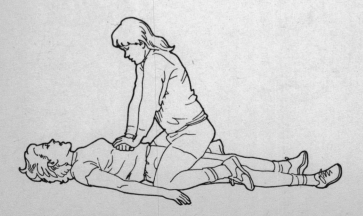

If you are alone and choking: Use your fist to perform the maneuver on yourself, placing the thumb-side of the fist of one hand against the abdomen just above the navel and grasping the fist with the other hand. Or try anything that will apply upward force just below your diaphragm and above the navel. Lean forward and press into the edge of a table, the kitchen sink, or the back of a chair, for example (see illustration below).

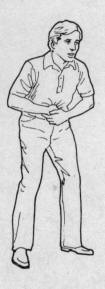

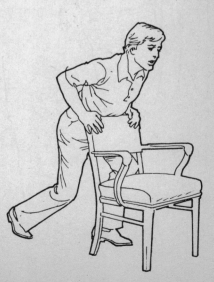

If the choking victim is overly fat and it is impossible to apply the abdominal thrust, or if the victim is in advanced pregnancy, use these measures:

Position yourself at one side and just behind the victim. Supporting the person with one hand on the breastbone, give four quick, forceful slaps with the heel of your other hand on the center of the back between the shoulder blades (see illustration below).

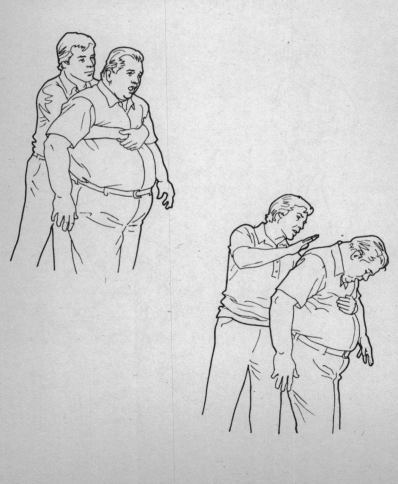

If this fails to dislodge the obstruction, use the chest thrust: Stand behind the victim and place the thumb-side of your fist high on the chest (about armpit level) in the *middle* of the breastbone, *not on the ribs*. Taking care not to squeeze the chest, grasp your fist with your other hand and, with your forearms, make four quick backward movements (see illustration, page 272).

If an Infant is Choking, use the following technique, recommended by the American Academy of Pediatrics.*

(*Caution:* Don't apply any measures if the child can breathe, speak or make sounds, and is coughing. These signs mean he is getting air in his windpipe that can expel the object partially blocking his airway. Any maneuvers by you interfere with this natural process and may convert the partial blockage to a total obstruction. *Watch closely but don't interfere*.)

If the choking infant is unable to breathe or make a sound, place the baby face down over your forearm (with the infant's head lower than the rest of his body). Using the heel of your hand, give four forceful but measured blows (less hard than for an adult) on the baby's back between the shoulder blades (see illustration below).

*Based on official statements published in Pediatrics, May and July 1982 © 1981, 1982 by the American Academy of Pediatrics.

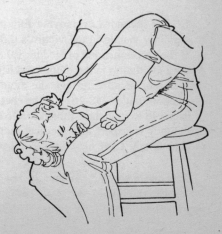

If the back blow fails to eject the object from the windpipe, apply four rapid chest thrusts. To do this: Turn the baby over on his back. Position him on your thighs with his head lower than his torso (as in illustration). *Using only the index and middle fingers of one hand*, place your fingers on the center of the baby's chest at the level of the nipples, *and compress the chest, as in CPR, four times in rapid succession* (see below).

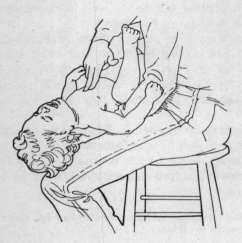

Do not attempt to remove a foreign body with your fingers unless it is plainly visible in the victim's throat.

If the recommended procedure is not successful, open the airway by placing the thumb in the mouth and lifting the lower jaw forward. Then deliver four breaths through the mouth or mouth-nose (as in artificial respiration, pages 258-261). If the chest fails to rise, repeat the sequence of back blows and chest thrusts while having someone call for help and emergency transport to a medical facility or for a rescue unit to come to your home. CPR may be necessary (see page 263).

Preparedness Note: If you are the parent of a young child, discuss the subject of choking with your pediatrician. Ask the physician to show you just how much force to use with the backslap and the chest thrust.

Because no single first-aid measure for choking works every time or in all circumstances, highly respected policy-making groups in the medical field advise beginning the rescue of the choking victim with four quick slaps with the heel of the hand on the victim's back between the shoulder blades. If this doesn't work, they advise, quickly apply the Heimlich Maneuver (the abdominal thrust). Proponents of the maneuver recommend, however, that if you are certain the person is choking, the technique should be applied at once—without delay for back blows or other anti-choking measures.

COLD—OVEREXPOSURE, FROSTBITE

Overexposure (Hypothermia): The symptoms include: numbness, drowsiness, staggering, failing vision, unconsciousness. If the person is unconscious, wrap him in blankets, call an ambulance or take him to the nearest hospital emergency facility at once. Watch breathing—and apply artificial respiration if necessary (see page 258). If the victim is conscious, place him in a warm room and wrap in blankets. Give warm, *non-alcoholic* drinks. Summon medical help.

Frostbite: Just before frostbite occurs, the victim's skin may be flushed; but, as the condition develops, the skin may turn white or gray-yellow. Often there is no pain, only numbness or tingling. *Do not rub the frozen members or apply snow*. Bring the victim indoors as soon as possible.

The best treatment for frostbite is rapid rewarming of the affected area. Immerse the frozen part in a warm—*but not hot*—bath. The temperature should be between 104 and 108 degrees F. (40–42° C.) Use an oral thermometer to test it. Discontinue warming as soon as the part becomes flushed.

CUTS, SCRATCHES, ABRASIONS

1. To minimize the possibility of infection, wash your hands thoroughly before treating any wound. Clean the skin around the wound with soap and water. To avoid contamination, wash away from the wound, not toward it.

2. Then, wash the wound itself with soap, flush it thoroughly with water and gently pat dry.

3. Cover the wound with sterile gauze, or the cleanest cloth available, held in place by bandage or adhesive tape.

4. Remember that with any wound there is always danger of tetanus (lockjaw); in deep, extensive or dirty wounds, the threat is serious. Try to find out whether the victim has been previously immunized with tetanus toxoid and whether immunity has been maintained with booster shots, so that the doctor can determine proper treatment.

5. Watch carefully for these signs of infection (which may not appear for several days): (a) a reddened, hot, painful area surrounding the wound; (b) red streaks radiating from the wound up the arm or leg; (c) swelling around the wound, accompanied by chills or fever. If infection should appear, see a doctor at once.

DIABETIC COMA AND INSULIN REACTION

IF SOMEONE BECOMES CONFUSED, incoherent or unconscious for no apparent reason, he may be a diabetic who is having an insulin reaction or developing a diabetic coma.

Insulin reaction is the result of a too-rapid drop in the diabetic's blood-sugar level. Symptoms come on rapidly. The diabetic sweats profusely and is nervous; his pulse is rapid, his breathing shallow. He may be hazy and faltering. If he is conscious and can swallow, give him some form of sugar—candy, lump sugar, fruit juice or a sweet soft drink. If recovery is not prompt, or if the diabetic cannot swallow, or is unconscious, summon a physician or ambulance and take the person immediately to the nearest emergency medical facility.

The symptoms of diabetic coma come on gradually. The diabetic's skin becomes flushed and dry, tongue dry, behavior drowsy, breathing labored; breath develops a fruity odor (like nail-polish remover). Diabetic coma requires prompt medical attention and emergency hospitalization.

DISLOCATED JOINTS

DO NOT ATTEMPT TO move the joint or set the dislocation yourself. Get medical attention promptly. If you must move the victim, first use splints to immobilize the joint in the position in which you found it. If the person has a hip dislocation, call an ambulance or move him on a stretcher to a hospital emergency room. To reduce swelling and relieve pain, apply an insulated ice bag to the injured part.

DROWNING

IF THE VICTIM is not breathing, clear the airway and start mouth-to-mouth respiration at once (see page 258). Administer CPR if the heart has stopped (see page 261). Take special precautions if broken neck is suspected (see page 265).

ELECTRIC SHOCK

EVERY SECOND of contact with the source of electricity lessens the victim's chance of survival. Break the victim's contact with the source of current in the quickest safe way possible. Indoors, disconnect the plug of the offending appliance, or pull the main switch at the fuse box. Outdoors, use a *dry* pole or branch.

Remove body from contact with current, using a dry, nonmetallic pole, a dry rope or dry clothing to push or pull the wire off the victim— or the victim off the wire. Stand on a dry surface, and touch only dry, nonconductive materials. Don't touch the victim until contact with current has been broken. Then check to see if the victim is breathing and has a pulse. If necessary, administer mouth-to-mouth breathing (see page 258) or CPR (see page 261). Send for medical aid at once. Check for burns or wounds at the current's entry and exit points.

If it is necessary to move the victim again, check to be sure the accident has not caused bone fractures or internal injuries. (See "Moving an Injured Person," page 282.)

EPILEPTIC SEIZURE, CONVULSION

IF POSSIBLE, turn the person having a seizure on one side. Don't try to restrain convulsive movement. Move furniture or nearby objects that might cause injury while the person is making involuntary movements. *Don't put anything in the person's mouth*. The seizure usually ends within a few minutes. When it ends, the person may experience some confusion. Reassure him and offer any assistance needed. If the spasms last longer than ten minutes, call a physician.

EYE—SOMETHING IN

FIRST, EXAMINE THE EYE by pulling down the lower lid and turning back the upper lid. If the speck is on either lid, try to remove it by touching it lightly with the corner of a clean cloth. If the speck is on the eye itself, don't attempt to remove it. Place a bandage over both eyes and take the person to a doctor.

FAINTING

PLACE THE PERSON ON HIS BACK. Make certain that his airway is clear and that he is breathing. Loosen tight clothing; apply cold cloths to his face.

If the fainting lasts more than a minute or two, keep him covered, if necessary to maintain normal body temperature, and call an ambulance or take him to a hospital emergency facility.

Fainting may be caused by fatigue, hunger, sudden emotional upset, a poorly ventilated room, etc. The person's breathing is usually weak, pulse feeble, face pale and the forehead covered with beads of perspiration. If the person merely feels faint, have him lie down.

HEAD INJURY—FRACTURE, CONCUSSION

THERE IS THE POSSIBILITY of head injury in any traffic accident, fall or other incident of violence. Symptoms may include: victim dazed or unconscious; rapid but weak pulse; bleeding from mouth, nose or ears (if there is much bleeding, pulse may be slow); pupils of eyes unequal in size; paralysis of one or more extremities; headache or dizziness; double vision; vomiting; pallor. Or the victim may appear quite normal and have a momentary loss of consciousness or a lack of memory of the event causing the injury—only to lapse into unconsciousness later, or to develop the other symptoms.

If the victim is unconscious, check breathing and pulse. Perform mouth-to-mouth respiration (see page 258) or CPR (see page 261) if necessary. If these steps are not needed and no neck or back injury is suspected, turn the victim on his side so that blood or mucus can drain from the corner of the mouth. Get medical assistance at once.

Even though the blow may not have brought unconsciousness, there is always danger of brain hemorrhage and serious trouble later. Lying quietly lessens the chance of hemorrhage. If the scalp is bleeding, place a dressing over the wound and bandage it into place. Keep the patient lying down until you get medical help or can deliver him to a hospital emergency facility.

HEART ATTACK

COMMON SYMPTOMS of heart attack are extreme shortness of breath, nausea, anxiety, pain in the center of the chest, sometimes radiating into the neck or arms, or occasionally pain in the upper abdomen. The patient may sweat and lose consciousness.

Do not ignore the symptoms of a heart attack. Call for emergency medical assistance at once. If the patient is having trouble breathing, do not force him to lie down. Help him take the position that is most comfortable for him. Loosen tight clothing (belt, collar, etc.). Don't attempt to lift or carry him. Don't give him anything to drink. Remain calm, and try to reassure him. Rehearse in your mind the steps in CPR (see page 261), in case the patient loses his pulse and stops breathing.

HEAT STROKE—HEAT EXHAUSTION

THE VICTIM of heat stroke is weak, irritable, dazed, nauseated. Sweating stops; skin becomes hot, red and dry. Temperature soars—maybe to

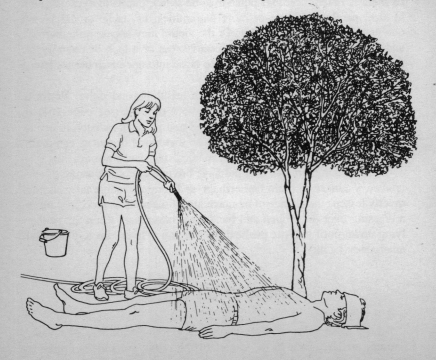

105° F. (40.5° C.) or higher, and the victim may lose consciousness.

Heat stroke is a life-threatening condition. Place the victim in a shaded place and cool him off as quickly as possible. Use a garden hose—running water is an ideal cooling method. If no hose is available, pour cool water over the victim—buckets of it. Or wrap his head in cold, wet towels and his body in a cold, wet sheet (see illustration page 280). If the person is conscious, give cool drinks but no stimulants. Cooling is the first step, but call an ambulance. Get the victim of heat stroke to a hospital emergency facility as quickly as possible.

Heat exhaustion (headache, extreme fatigue, dizziness, cold, clammy and pale skin, perhaps fainting—but normal or only slightly elevated temperature) can be treated by rest in a shaded area or air-conditioned room.

Have the person lie down with legs and feet raised 8 to 12 inches higher than the level of his head. Place cold towels on his head, but avoid chilling. Give sips of cool, diluted salt water—one teaspoon salt (5 grams) to one 8-oz. glass (236 ml.) of water—at the rate of half a glass every 15 minutes for an hour. Orange juice is helpful. If the victim becomes nauseated, don't give more fluids. Take him to the nearest emergency facility.

HYPERVENTILATION

HYPERVENTILATION is a common complication of emotional upset and most often affects anxious, high-strung persons who unknowingly breathe too rapidly. This disturbs the normal balance of carbon dioxide in the blood. The result is tingling and spasms of the fingers and toes and a peculiar numbness around the mouth. These symptoms make the victim still more anxious, and still more hyperventilation results. The patient's color and pulse remain good.

Not a dangerous condition, hyperventilation can usually be helped by reassurance and this simple measure: Have the person breathe slowly for ten minutes, occasionally longer, into a paper (not plastic) bag held tightly over his mouth and nose. If this does not work, take the patient to a hospital emergency facility.

MOVING AN INJURED PERSON

IF AN INJURY involves the neck or back, damage can be done by moving the victim. Get a doctor or ambulance quickly, if possible; meanwhile, cover the patient with blankets or coats if necessary to maintain body temperature. Don't attempt to change his position until you determine the nature of his injuries—unless moving is absolutely necessary to prevent further injuries. If the victim must be pulled to safety, move his body lengthwise (*not sidewise*) and *head first*, with his head and neck carefully supported. If possible, slip a blanket or long coat under him so he can ride on that (see illustration below). If the person must be lifted, don't jackknife him by lifting his heels and head only. Support each part of the body so that you lift it in a straight line as if the person were lying on a board.

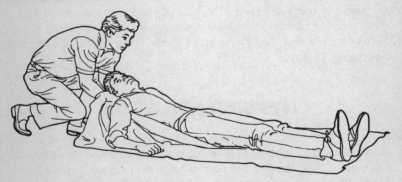

Until you are certain that there is no neck or back injury, don't bundle a seriously injured person into an automobile and speed to the nearest town. If a victim must be transported, move him in a reclining or semi-reclining position. Improvise a stretcher, if possible. The most desirable is a door or wide board. Lacking either of these, make a stretcher out of blankets and poles, or out of buttoned jackets with the sleeves turned inward and the poles run through the sleeves. If the victim is conscious, and not suffering from back, neck or leg injuries, use a chair (carried by two or more persons) to bring him down narrow or winding stairs.

When reporting an accident, inform the doctor or ambulance service of the nature of the accident and injuries. Seek advice regarding the safest procedure.

NOSE—SOMETHING IN

IF THE OBJECT cannot be withdrawn easily, consult a doctor at once. Don't permit violent nose-blowing. Don't probe the nose yourself; you may push the object deeper or injure the nostril.

NOSEBLEED

HAVE THE PATIENT pinch the fleshy part of the nose and sit quietly with head inclined forward for 15 minutes. This may cause a clot to form over the ruptured blood vessels.

If the bleeding continues, pack each bleeding nostril with a plug of sterile gauze. Be careful to leave one end of each plug outside so that it can be easily removed. Have the patient lie down, with his head elevated, and place a cold, wet towel across his face. Recurrent nosebleed should have medical attention.

POISON IVY, OAK, SUMAC

WASH EXPOSED AREAS with soap and cold water as soon as possible, working up a thick lather and rinsing several times. *Do not scrub with a brush*. If itching and burning have already appeared, wash the affected areas gently with soap and cold water, and pat on calamine lotion to soothe the itch. If you are frequently or seriously bothered by poison ivy, ask your doctor about the possibility of immunization.

POISONING, BY MOUTH

CALL YOUR POISON CONTROL CENTER or your doctor immediately. Tell what the suspected poison is and follow instructions.

- If you can't get medical aid, or the poison is unknown, dilute the poison in the stomach by giving the victim two or three cups (472 to 708 ml.) of water. (If the victim is a child under five years old, give one cup—236 ml.—of water.) *Don't induce vomiting*.

- *Don't induce vomiting* if the victim has swallowed a corrosive poison such as carbolic acid, toilet bowl cleaner, lye, drain cleaner, ammonia, or a volatile substance such as kerosene or gasoline. Instead, dilute the poison in the victim's stomach:

Give one cup (236 ml.) of water for a child under five years old. Give one to two cups (236 to 472 ml.) of water if the victim is over five. Get the victim to the hospital emergency facility at once. Always take the poison container with you.

Caution: Never attempt to administer fluids if the victim is asleep or is having a convulsion. Call for emergency medical help, or the ambulance to take him to the hospital at once.

- If the swallowed poison is neither a corrosive nor a volatile substance (and the victim is not asleep or having a convulsion), *induce the victim to vomit*.

For a child one to five years old give one tablespoon (15 ml.) of syrup of ipecac followed by one to two cups (236 to 472 ml.) of water. If the victim is five years old or older, give one to two tablespoons (15 to 30 ml.) of syrup of ipecac, followed by one to two cups (236 to 472 ml.) of water. If no vomiting occurs in 20 minutes, the dose *may be repeated once only*.

- If the powdered activated charcoal is available, give the powder mixed in water. Use the amounts recommended on the package. This material will take up large quantities of the ingested poison and conduct it through the intestinal tract. Activated charcoal will also deactivate syrup of ipecac, so, if the latter is used, *give charcoal only after the ipecac has induced vomiting*.

● If the antidotes recommended above are not available, give several glasses of water and stick your finger into the victim's throat.

PUNCTURE WOUNDS

1. Wash your hands, then clean the wound with soap and water.
2. Cover the wound loosely with a sterile dressing. Apply an insulated ice bag to reduce swelling, relieve pain, and slow absorption of toxicity.
3. Take the patient to a doctor or a hospital emergency facility. The doctor will clean the wound, opening it further if necessary, and will take steps to protect against tetanus.

SHOCK—HOW TO TREAT IT

IN ANY SERIOUS INJURY (such as bleeding wound, fracture, major burn), always expect shock, and act to lessen it. The symptoms: the skin is pale, cold and clammy; the pulse is rapid; breathing is shallow, rapid or irregular; the injured person is frightened, restless, apprehensive or comatose.

1. Keep the patient lying down. In cases of head or chest injuries, when the patient has difficulty breathing, the head and shoulders should be raised so that the head is ten inches higher than the feet.
2. Maintain normal body temperature.
3. Loosen any restrictive clothing and keep the person as calm and comfortable as possible.
4. Get the patient to a hospital emergency facility, or call for emergency medical assistance.

SPLINTERS

WASH YOUR HANDS and the skin around the splinter with soap and water. Sterilize a needle and tweezers by boiling them in water or by heating them in the flame of a match and wiping off the carbon with sterile gauze. Loosen the skin around the splinter with the needle, and remove splinter with the tweezers. If the splinter breaks or is lodged deeply, see a doctor.

SPRAINS

ELEVATE THE INJURED JOINT to a comfortable position and prevent further movement. Persons with an affected knee or ankle should not be allowed to walk. Apply an insulated ice bag or a cold compress over the sprain to reduce pain and swelling. Sprains should be examined by a doctor for possible bone fracture.

STINGS—BEE, WASP, HORNET

IN THE CASE OF A BEE STING, try to remove the stinger and venom sac by gently scraping with a sterilized knife. Run cold water over and around the sting to relieve pain and slow the absorption of the venom, or place an insulated ice bag over it. Calamine lotion may relieve itching.

Soak a victim of massive stings (by a swarm of insects) in a cold bath in which baking soda has been dissolved. Use one tablespoon (14 grams) of baking soda per quart (1 liter of water). An allergic person reacts violently to insect stings; he should be taken promptly to the nearest hospital emergency room. Any person who is allergic should ask the physician to prescribe an anti-insect sting kit and should keep it always on hand. (Kits not available without prescription.)

STINGS AND BITES— POISONOUS SPIDERS AND SCORPION

KEEP THE VICTIM lying quietly and maintain normal body temperature. There may be a redness and swelling around the sting, along with painful abdominal or muscle cramps, fever, sweating and nausea. A tingling or burning pain may spread through the body.

Pack ice wrapped in cloth around the wound to slow the spread of the poison. (The U.S. tarantula is not seriously poisonous, but its bite is painful and can cause bacterial infection.) Summon a doctor or take the patient to a hospital emergency facility.

STOMACH PAIN—APPENDICITIS

DO NOT GIVE the patient a laxative. Take his temperature. Feel his abdomen while he is lying down with his abdominal muscles relaxed. If there is any fever, even slight, and if the abdomen feels hard or tense and is sore or painful to the touch, especially on the lower right side, call a doctor at once or take the patient to a hospital emergency room. The trouble may be appendicitis. Other appendicitis symptoms: nausea, vomiting, persistent pain. When there is pain in the lower right side of the abdomen, suspect appendicitis until another diagnosis is proved. Meanwhile, don't let the patient eat anything; food or a laxative increases the possibility of the appendix rupturing. Don't let him drink anything.

SUNBURN

IF THE SKIN is reddened but not blistered, apply cold wet compresses to the sunburned area to alleviate pain, or submerge the area in cold water. Do not use butter or margarine; either may irritate or introduce infection. If the skin is blistered or extensively burned, cover it with a cloth wet with cold water. Severe or extensive sunburn requires prompt medical aid. Do not re-expose sunburned skin until healing is complete.

SWALLOWED OBJECTS

SMALL, ROUND OBJECTS (beads, buttons, coins, marbles) swallowed by children usually pass uneventfully through the intestines and are eliminated. Do not give cathartics or bulky foods—just the normal diet.

If there is pain, or if the child develops a cough, consult a doctor.

Sharp or straight objects (bobby pins, open safety pins, bones) are dangerous. Don't panic; consult a doctor. Special instruments may be required to locate and remove the object.

THROAT—SOMETHING CAUGHT IN

IF SOMETHING is caught in the throat (pharynx), it may obstruct swallowing or breathing or both. If only swallowing is obstructed, the person should proceed as calmly as possible to the nearest hospital emergency facility.

If the object plugs the airway, treat for choking (see page 268).

UNCONSCIOUSNESS—CAUSE UNKNOWN

IF YOU ENCOUNTER an unconscious person, and the nature of the trouble is unknown: (1) Open the airway (see page 258). (2) If the victim is not breathing or is breathing with great difficulty, apply artificial respiration (see page 258). If his pulse has stopped, apply cardiopulmonary resuscitation (see page 261). (3) Check for emergency medical identification, perhaps a card stating that the victim is a diabetic (see page 276) or an epileptic or has some other specific illness. (4) If the victim's face is pale, pulse weak, lower his head slightly. (5) If his lips are blue, check his breathing and pulse. Apply artificial respiration or CPR if necessary. (6) If an unconscious person vomits, to prevent choking turn him on his side if his neck is not broken. (7) Get as full a report as possible as to what happened; ask everyone present.

Have someone call an ambulance. Do not move victim unless absolutely necessary to prevent further harm. (see "Moving an Injured Person," page 282.) Do not disturb or remove an unconscious stranger's personal effects, or anything that may be evidence of a crime or attempted suicide, unless it is clearly essential to save the person's life. *Remember:* Never give fluids to an unconscious person.

WARNING

DISCARD OLD DRUGS AND KEEP OTHERS LOCKED UP

REMEMBER that drugs do not last indefinitely. They may lose their potency, evaporate to harmful concentrations, or their components may recombine harmfully.

To prevent deterioration, keep all bottles tightly stoppered. Keep medicines in a cool, dry, preferably dark place.

Discard as unsafe any preparation that has changed color or consistency or become cloudy. Especially avoid the use of old iodine, eye drops, eye washes, nose drops, cough remedies, ointments.

Keep all medications, including nonprescription drugs such as aspirin, out of reach of children. When discarding drugs, be sure to dispose of them where they cannot be retrieved by children or pets.

FIRST-AID KIT

ASSEMBLE YOUR FIRST-AID SUPPLIES *now*, before you need them. Tailor the contents to fit your family's particular needs. Don't add first-aid supplies to the jumble of toothpaste and cosmetics in the medicine cabinet. Instead, assemble them in a suitably labeled box (such as a fishing-tackle box or small tool chest with hinged cover), so that everything will be handy when needed. Label everything in the kit clearly, and indicate what it is used for. Put in a copy of this handbook.

Be sure not to lock the box—otherwise you may be hunting for the key when seconds count. Place the box on a shelf beyond the reach of small children. Check it periodically and always restock items as soon as they are used up.

CHECKLIST OF SUPPLIES

(All items except anti-sting kit are obtainable without prescription.)

Sterile gauze dressing, 4 × 4 inches (10 × 10 cm.) individually wrapped, for cleaning and covering wounds.

. Roll of gauze bandage, 2 inches wide (5 cm.), for bandaging sterile dressings over wounds, etc.

Three squares of cloth 42 × 42 inches (107 × 107 cm.) for triangular bandages and slings. Supply of safety pins 1½ inches (4 cm.) long.

Box of assorted adhesive dressings (Band-Aid, Curad, or similar products).

Roll of inch-wide (2½ cm.) adhesive tape.

Roll of absorbent cotton.

Pint bottle of sterile saline solution—one level teaspoonful (5 grams) of salt to one pint (472 ml.) of boiled water.

Tube of petroleum jelly.

Bottle of calamine lotion, for sunburn, insect bites, rashes, etc.

Bottle of ipecac syrup to induce vomiting.

Container of powdered, activated charcoal to deactivate swallowed poisons.

Box of baking soda (bicarbonate of soda).

Pair of scissors.

Pair of tweezers.

Packet of needles.

Sharp knife or packet of stiff-backed razor blades.

Medicine (eye) dropper.

Measuring cup.

Oral thermometer.

Rectal thermometer.

Hot-water bottle.

Ice bag.

Box of wooden safety matches.

Flashlight.

Coins (for pay phone when you take the kit with you on motor trips).

EMERGENCY TELEPHONE NUMBERS

In many areas, one telephone number will activate the community's emergency medical system. In some communities the number is that of the police department. Find out what the number is in your town and insert it prominently in the list below.

AMBULANCE_____
Phone

DOCTOR_____
Phone

DOCTOR_____
Phone

HOSPITAL EMERGENCY FACILITY_____
Phone

POLICE DEPARTMENT_____
Phone

FIRE DEPARTMENT_____
Phone

24-HOUR PHARMACY_____
Phone

NEIGHBORHOOD PHARMACY_____
Phone

ELECTRIC COMPANY_____
Phone

GAS COMPANY_____
Phone

OTHER NUMBERS:_____

_____

_____

_____

_____

_____